D0379301

Praise

"Bailey Gaddis brings a fresh new approach to holistic prenatal preparation in this uplifting and reassuring book that draws from the harmonizing principles of feng shui. It's an engaging read that takes your mind on a gentle trip down a river of wisdom, inspiring you to practice self-care and enjoy personal growth throughout the childbearing year."

— **Pam England**, author of *Birthing from Within*

"With wisdom, wit, and honesty, Bailey Gaddis offers mothers heartfelt advice that is as fresh as it is insightful. Bailey leads readers through a new, wonderful journey toward motherhood. If you're pregnant, 'just breathe,' and read this book!"

— **Robin Gerber**, author of *Leadership the Eleanor Roosevelt Way*

"Bailey Gaddis has a beautiful and magnetic gift for allowing women to make much-needed shifts within themselves in a fun, spirited, and interesting way. Her approach is holistic yet entertaining, deep yet relatable, and it makes you laugh out loud while you tackle the big changes and fears pregnancy brings. In this book Bailey teaches women how to care for themselves on all levels, and she allows them to easily and effectively step into the enormous sea of transformation of pregnancy and motherhood. This book is like having a trusted and wise sister to hold your hand and tell you everything you need to know as you embark on this journey."

— **Taryn Longo**, transformational teacher for women and founder and director of Wild Heart Mama

"This book is very well written and easy to read, with excellent ideas to make your birth experience the best it can be. Every birth experience is unique; childbirth is primal, and your experience is influenced by your culture. Fear of the unknown makes the experience worse, and preparation makes all the difference. Being open to what you and your baby need will make your experience better. The goal of every delivery is a healthy mom and healthy baby. This guide is a tool that may help you find balance and comfort in your life overall, not only in childbirth."

— **Kristi Schoeld, MD**

"We love Bailey Gaddis's sense of humor and authenticity throughout the book! This is such a great tool for mamas who want to be empowered, and it can lead them to have a more magical birth than they thought possible. Bailey is a gifted teacher and an incredible, essential part of any birth."
— **Rebecca and Josh Tickell**, Sundance Award–winning filmmakers and founders of Big Picture Ranch

"As the saying goes, 'Even mothers need to be mothered,' and *Feng Shui Mommy* mastermind Bailey Gaddis, in her refreshingly authentic and honest, inherently trustworthy voice, does just that. Like a long-lost best friend, she creates a welcoming, nourishing oasis of safety, empowerment, and support for new mothers. She seamlessly weaves practical yet profound, ever-reassuring, often hilarious, and absolutely indispensable pregnancy and birthing wisdom with nurturing, uplifting food for the soul and spirit: the perfect recipe for a healthy, healing, joyful experience of pregnancy, birth, and motherhood. Bailey's gloriously grounded approach and her normalizing of pregnancy, birth, and motherhood elevate the experience to its rightful place as a spiritual milestone and the transformational opportunity of every woman's lifetime to step into her truest, richest, and most resplendent, liberated self: balanced, confident, powerful, harmonious, and whole — the Feng Shui Mommy! This delightful, inspiring book had my ovaries popping, my oxytocin pumping, and my heart champing at the bit to embark on the awesome, miraculous magic-carpet ride of mommyhood all over again!"

— **Jessica Cauffiel**, actor, writer, producer, shaman

"Meet Bailey Gaddis, the fresh-voiced, bright-eyed, fully engaged mama mystic whose knowledge and passion for helping mothers find their bliss before, during, and after pregnancy are truly inspiring. A book brimming with fabulous resources, humor, and beautiful reflections, *Feng Shui Mommy* will be a favorite companion for your journey to motherhood and beyond."
— **Zhena Muzyka**, author of *Life by the Cup* and publisher of Enliven Books

FENG SHUI
MOMMY

FENG SHUI
MOMMY

CREATING BALANCE *and* HARMONY
for BLISSFUL PREGNANCY,
CHILDBIRTH, *and* MOTHERHOOD

BAILEY GADDIS

New World Library
Novato, California

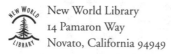

New World Library
14 Pamaron Way
Novato, California 94949

Copyright © 2017 by Bailey Gaddis

All rights reserved. This book may not be reproduced in whole or in part, stored in a retrieval system, or transmitted in any form or by any means — electronic, mechanical, or other — without written permission from the publisher, except by a reviewer, who may quote brief passages in a review.

The material in this book is intended for education. It is not meant to take the place of diagnosis and treatment by a qualified medical practitioner or therapist. No expressed or implied guarantee of the effects of the use of the recommendations can be given or liability taken.

Illustrations by Amanda Sandoval
Text design by Tona Pearce Myers

Library of Congress Cataloging-in-Publication data is available.

First printing, May 2017
ISBN 978-1-60868-471-7
Ebook ISBN 978-1-60868-472-4

Printed in Canada on 100% postconsumer-waste recycled paper

New World Library is proud to be a Gold Certified Environmentally Responsible Publisher. Publisher certification awarded by Green Press Initiative. www.greenpressinitiative.org

10   9   8   7   6   5   4   3   2

To my son, Hudson, for waking up a better version of my Self, and to my partner, Eric, for being my cocaptain through the nitty-gritty of parenthood. You boys rock.

Birth is not only about making babies. It's about making mothers — strong, competent, capable mothers who trust themselves and know their inner strength.

— *Barbara Katz Rothman*

CONTENTS

MY PREGNANCY AND
BIRTH STORY

JUST BREATHE: *Inhale to a slow count of eight, hold for a count of two, and exhale to a slow count of eight. Repeat until you settle into a deep and rhythmic breathing pattern. As you read, return to this breath and allow it to calm you if any part of this story triggers an emotion you would like to melt away. Each pregnancy and birth story you encounter will be unique to the individual telling it: absorb the pieces of the story that inspire you and allow the rest to stay with the teller. Your experience will be your own.*

There once was a super sperm, stronger than all the rest, who found its way into the loving caress of a waiting egg. Together they bonded, creating a miracle as profound as the birth of a star, or a baby sleeping through the night. This blooming miracle began to grow in size, and its carrier vessel expanded to accommodate it. As the vessel expanded, her outer coverings began to stretch, her bosom swelled, and her flatulence became uncontrollable. Magic was happening.

The week before I peed on "the stick to end all sticks," my partner, Eric, and I were suffering from paralyzing indecision over which summer concerts to go to and whether we should toy around with going vegan (we didn't).

Our indecisive paralysis shifted into more of a catatonic meltdown when we found out what excellent decision makers our sperm and egg were.

Who knew that a tiny pink symbol on a pee-soaked stick could render you mute and useless for twenty-four hours? And what a transformation! In that time I went from a champagne-sipping, coffee-coddling, carefree woman to a "the smell of your mimosa makes me nauseous, and the coffee you're able to sip makes me want to cry" future mother. It's glorious! Really, it is. People carry your groceries.

The dainty tower of mind-body-spirit alignment I had been so meticulously piecing together was blown down in one mighty gush of the bladder. Saying I was afraid of the changes that come with pregnancy doesn't begin to cover it. Those two pink lines sent multiple blasts of shock through me and awakened so much darkness — denial, confusion, loss, nausea, selfishness... Mixed with the dark was a welcome blend of bliss and excitement. Who knew there was enough space for it all!

Although the water in the pregnancy pond was not ideal, climbing out of it was not an option. I was in my late twenties and in a new but committed relationship, I had a sad yet stable bank account, and most importantly, I *felt* that the pregnancy was right. It was like my spirit had popped its head up and slapped the Nike slogan on my forehead.

Though I was terrified of "just doing it," I still had a strange compulsion to tell everyone about my unplanned pregnancy, because early pregnancy hormones made me emotionally masochistic. News of my sans-wedlock pregnancy made the ladies at my grandparent's Catholic retirement center say "Huh?" (and start praying), and made my New Age Mama friends say, "Welcome to the club. Will you be eating your placenta?"

My perspective on the situation shifted every five to ten minutes during the first few weeks after "the Urination." One minute I would be miserably dry-heaving in the toilet (because that's what pregnant women do, right?), and seven minutes later I would be joyfully wolfing down a foot-long sub (because that's what pregnant women do, right?). I was a hot mess. No, really — I was *so* hot.

There wasn't a magic pill to quell my craziness. I just had to allow myself to be a multiple-personality pregnant lady until I figured out how to settle into my new reality. To begin the process of settling in, I flipped into my type A "get shift done" mode. I made more long sandwiches, and I made lists. Lots of lists.

Because just about every aspect of my identity in the world was suddenly up for grabs, I made a list for each of the core elements of my life: romantic relationship, family, friends, career, body, spirit, home, neurosis over anything I don't control — you know, the normal stuff. On each list I brainstormed about how my journey into motherhood would affect that element of life, and how I would spend the next seven-ish months preparing for (or releasing my resistance to) those effects. I also made lists for Eric. He was totally into it.

I then took one item from one list every day, and did it. Pregnancy got easier after that; I fell into something that didn't quite resemble a *groove* but was more like a trough, which presumably led to childbirth.

Spoiler Alert: The Baby Made It Out

Did you know the birthing body can bust through hundreds of brick walls with the serenity of a monk melting ice with his mind?

My inner control freak was knocked off her throne when my son was not born on the date my doctor marked on his shipping slip. No one had told me that only 5 percent of babies are born on their due date. My sham due date of June 19 ostentatiously arrived, and then flitted away with no baby — at least not my baby. I was irked (totally pissed), convinced my child was going to live in my womb forever, content to nuzzle my bladder, jab my ribs, and spawn a lifetime of constipation. The only excitement on this Day That Was Not *The* Day was a few bouts of irritable bowel. An "overdue" pregnant woman likely coined the phrase "adding insult to injury."

Another twenty-four hours passed, and that now-frazzled control freak in me totally panicked. All semblance of control was lost. I had sex, shuffled four miles, doused my tomato juice with hot sauce, and found a YouTube "labor-inducing" video that required me to dance to the Tootsee Roll song. Nothing. "If shaking my rump to a nineties rap song won't do it, what will?"

Castor oil. Lube it up.

On June 21, I took three 1-teaspoon doses of castor oil. I have never seen any variety of oil since without the irrepressible urge to re-meet my last meal. I took my third dose at around 5:00 PM and waited for water to boil.

When Eric returned from work two hours later, I was ready to heap my last batch of coal on the baby train: Mexican food. Before we reached the salty crumbs of our first basket of chips, my bowels lashed out. I rushed to the bathroom, expecting mayhem; nothing happened. After an additional bathroom visit provided no number two, I suspected something was up, or coming down, and that we'd better get the check and get the heck out of there. I had no desire to deliver my baby on the grungy floor of a Mexican restaurant bathroom, alongside a dusty antique crucifix.

After being graced with one more "urge for an internal purge" on our way home, followed by nothing, I got into bed and began watching a chick flick about a woman who's been implanted with the wrong man's sperm. One hour later *everything* began tightening, cramping, and surging, without going out for recess. (My hair even tightened; I swear it's been curlier since going through childbirth.) I started to fear that castor oil was more malicious than mischievous.

"If I'm having contractions, aren't they supposed to be in perfectly timed intervals? Aren't there supposed to be breaks where I can eat ice cream and watch another movie? What the heck is up with this incessant tsunami?"

After pacing the four feet of my bathroom for a confusing hour, I woke up Eric with every expectant father's favorite words, "It's time." He called our doctor, who galvanized Eric into action when he spluttered the words "castor oil." Apparently, castor oil either produces unkind bowel movements or facilitates a speedy childbirth (because the contractions rarely break). Yay!

As soon as our Prius landed in a parking spot near the after-hours emergency room entrance, I allowed myself to go into the light — the light pouring from the "Off Limits" ambulance entrance. Someone yelled at me, then saw my belly.

I was in limbo for the first thirty minutes at the hospital, unsure if I was in labor but too consumed by physical sensations to care. Waves of energy reverberated from my uterus, causing tremors in my legs. The sensations were so far beyond pain they didn't even register as uncomfortable (we'll get into that phenomenon later). Because there was no room left for *me* amid the shaking, I floated above myself, observing the woman being racked by birth.

When a nurse confirmed that it was my uterus, not my bowels, causing all the commotion, a switch flipped and I allowed myself to fully check out of my body and into an ethereal space. As the birthing woman was wheeled to her labor and delivery room, I floated behind her, noticing the silent sounds of the time warp she was traveling through — leaving one world behind, and pushing into another.

I had spent months listening to guided meditation recordings that had me floating with unicorns and angels on rainbow-colored clouds of cotton candy. The scene my mind dropped me into during childbirth was much different. I found myself being sucked up into a behemoth wave as the surge of each contraction rolled through me, and I would reach the peak of the wall of water just as my body reached the peak of the surge. As the surge subsided I would slide down the back of the wave. Roughly thirty seconds would lapse before the next wave would draw me up.

Time ceased during my eleven-hour labor. All that spiritual (and now scientific) hubbub about time not actually existing became my perception of reality. Each surge was encapsulated in its own Twilight Zone. To allow this timeless state to persist, we closed the blinds, preventing the pervasive messages of the rising sun from intruding. Time did not cease for my doctor, however, who decided it was time to break my water. "It would speed things along."

This memory is like a shape-shifting dream that changes its story each time I try to remember it. Someone must have given consent for the intervention. Surely it wasn't me, but maybe it was. Maybe my doctor asked me while I was experiencing the peak of a surge. Maybe I so desperately wanted to meet my baby that I no longer cared how it happened. Maybe the doc just did it. I don't know, but I do know what it felt like as my baby juice (amniotic fluid) flowed out.

I felt emptiness. I felt like I was losing my padding. That liquid was the first product of labor to escape me, and its loss had impact. I could feel the (totally valid) possibility of my baby being born in-caul (and maybe becoming the next Dalai Lama) draining out of me. (Did you know Tibetan Buddhists seek Caulbearers to bring up to become potential Dalai Lamas?) I also felt relief that my baby might be coming sooner than expected — my labor was now hard.

And then I began to shift into the final phase of labor. The shift got real. I breathed through my nose, visualized my waves, and asked for an epidural.

Have you ever been in a rainstorm where you think, "Wow, it's raining really hard! It can't possibly rain any harder," and then it begins to rain harder? That's how my transition into the last act of labor was: really hard rain that was made of intense sensations and endorphins. I wasn't given the epidural. I was too far along (almost 9 cm dilated), and by the time I was pulled into another surge I forgot I had asked for it. Childbirth without an epidural was not easy, was worth every fierce moment, and gave me an insider's understanding of the reason some women choose to birth with drugs, and some without; they are *all* super rad mamas.

With each surge and purposeful breath, I was intent on giving my body the time it needed to gingerly ease my baby out. My doctor did not share my intent. I had visions of birth balls, squatting positions, and hip swirling to support my baby through emergence. My doctor did not share my visions. I received the classic hospital treatment: flat on my back, legs up in stirrups. Giddyup.

I was then instructed to "push!" for two hours. I now possess a cellular knowledge of the wall(s) that marathoners push through on the last leg of their journey — begging their body not to crumble, yet sure their mind (and spirit!) will carry them through. My eyes, unlike my perineum, remained closed during this final phase of labor, as animalistic grunts began erupting from somewhere in the room. ("Is that me?!") Childbirth is a great time to learn what your spirit animal is.

Next time around, I'll be gently breathing my baby down while floating in a warm pool of fairy water, as my birthing tribe hums sweet somethings into my ear — but I now realize that birth always has the potential to be incredible, regardless of the booby traps that may be wedged into the path (a.k.a. "a hospital bed with metal stirrups").

With a mighty (and surprisingly unpainful) push, Hudson's head materialized and my new life began. We did it! I did it! He did it! (And I didn't poop!)

My doctor slipped the remainder of the delicate little being out of my flummoxed womb and handed me a wailing piece of heaven. Euphoric warmth flooded me — an epic brand of love that spouted from my heart and poured into my core. Mama's Brand Love — so insane.

The birth of my son was far from what I expected and exactly what

I needed — an experience forged from a powerful alchemy of lioness-like strength, raw vulnerability, and unavoidable surrender. Up until the moment I first held my son I had secretly doubted my ability to do anything great in life, hiding my doubt behind a chipper face and a "sure thing!" attitude. But all doubts dissolved as the vulnerability, and the accompanying strength and surrender that were birthed with my baby, played in the light of my new life.

So what do you think? Ready to tap into your epic brand of love and sip from your cocktail of awesomeness? Let's start connecting you with your inner wisdom, and filling you with the knowledge and empowerment to create the journey into motherhood you were meant to have.

INTRODUCTION

This is the book I needed to read when I was pregnant. My pregnancy was unplanned, meaning I was not mentally (or physically, or spiritually) prepared for the swift kick in the uterus I got when the test registered positive. Before then, I thought I had been working a healthy, holistic lifestyle, but in reality, I was disconnected and disorganized in mind, body, and spirit. Getting pregnant was like a cosmic Feng Shui Master whispering loudly in my ear, "Get your energetic house in order, Bailey! You're really bad at being pregnant." She was right. If only I'd had this book — I would have been able to relax and let the various pieces of my life sort themselves out and shift into place. I would have enjoyed my pregnancy with a greater sense of authentic calm, even a sense of fun.

Three days after I peed on the stick, I ran out and bought thirty-five (mostly terrifying) books on pregnancy. The stack of books taunting me from the corner of our living room was enough to inject some serious fear into my early-days queasiness. I would pick up one of those books, begin to read, then snap the book shut when I reached a frightening cautionary tale, fell into a too-graphic description, or was confronted with a snooty, know-it-all narrative voice. These books, instead of nurturing me, kind of...scared the hell out of me.

But there was one book, a book on HypnoBirthing, that didn't freak me out. Instead, this book focused on the fact that if we could just quell our massive fears and anxieties and go inside to find trust in ourselves, we could have an untraumatic birth. I found myself drawn to this warm philosophy and the inclusive nature of the technique, which focused on the fact that what unites all of us soon-to-be mothers is that each of us will have our own unique experience. Heck, yeah!

That book helped me make contact with, and get really clear on, my own birthing desires. It also helped me get in touch with how out-of-whack the other parts of my life were. I found myself, in those early days, scrambling (internally and literally) to try to figure out how to be a loving romantic partner, keep my house clean, grow a healthy baby, not throw up every time I smelled seafood, and continue to work. So I knuckled down and got going, but not like I had in the past. Instead of running around from one mini-crisis to the next, I got into the business of working on *me*. Or, more specifically, I began to get to know myself in radically new ways. I began to get really clear about "all my stuff" — and to realize that my life was just too cluttered. Being pregnant was the push I needed to find my way to living in greater happy-truth and a more grounded place of integrity. So, along with birthing a baby, I also birthed my new Self (almost more challenging than the former).

I found I had a new calling, which was to become a certified Hypno-Birthing childbirth educator, birth doula, and hypnotherapist so I could support other women on this journey. Marrying these services with the professional organizing business I owned and my experience working in the in vitro fertilization industry allowed me to provide women with a comprehensive support system. My primary goal was to empower women to find their own birthing path — without feeling like it was "just hormones" in play when they found the power and peace of mind to politely tell the well-meaning birthing-opinionated stranger in the grocery store checkout line to mind her own cart.

This book unites all of my professional and deeply personal passions, with the intention of helping you create and hold as much space as you need to find your way into a state of blissful balance while you birth your baby and your new life.

How Feng Shui Fits In

What does feng shui have to do with your journey into motherhood? What does the term even mean?

Feng shui (pronounced "fung shway") is an ancient Chinese philosophy that focuses on harmonizing humans with our surrounding environment. Feng shui is based on the idea that nature, including our material environments, is alive with an invisible energy — our *chi*, or life force. In this book, the concept of feng shui is pushed beyond your physical environment into a space where your mental and spiritual environments, and the life force they're alive with, are honored.

This book offers support regarding how to nurture and harmonize the life force moving through these three primary aspects of your life — mental, physical, and spiritual — allowing you to move into childbirth and motherhood with a balanced, empowered, and calm energy and knowledge about how to realign that energy when it's knocked off balance. That's what being a Feng Shui Mommy is — knowing what it feels like to have balanced and harmonized life force flowing through all aspects of your existence, and knowing how to jump back into the flow when you've been thrown out.

How a Feng Shui Mommy
Expresses the Five Elements of Feng Shui

The philosophy of feng shui leans on the belief that energy, the life force of nature, lives in all things. Chi manifests into the physical world through water, wood, fire, earth, and metal — these elements must all interact to reproduce the pure and perfect state in which chi first enters this world. Kind of like the pure and perfect state of a new baby.

Chi cycles through the five elements by first arriving from the heavens via water. The water mixes with the earth and births plants (wood). The plants then feed the powerful energy of fire, dissolving into ash (earth). The ash turns into metal, and the cycle begins to repeat itself when metal attracts new water from the heavens.

The Feng Shui Mommy must move through a similar cycle to maintain harmony in her life — but her cycle will be expressed a bit differently.

She expresses her water element by removing one unneeded item from her physical space every day (to get the good energy flowing), and she creates fluidity in her mental space by pulling out all her to-dos and nagging thoughts and organizing them on paper (or on screen). Removing the stagnation of superfluous stuff from her physical and mental zones allows her spiritual world to become free flowing and ripe for exploration.

And she usually showers every day.

The nurturing of the Feng Shui Mommy's water element encourages the expression of her wood element, which she manifests through engaging in passions that combine the physical and spiritual for at least one hour a day. She may go to a yoga class, walk outside with the intent of receiving a special message from nature, support the growth of new life in a garden, or take a nap. (That's spiritual and physical, right? Maybe she can nap next to a Buddha sculpture.)

The growth of her wood element creates the fuel for her fire element to express itself through a daily block of time dedicated to her blend of creative expression (writing, painting, filming, sculpting, sketching, or maybe some cake decorating). And sex — she likes sex, even if she's by herself.

The energetic release the Feng Shui Mommy receives through the expression of her fire element allows her to settle into the stable support of her earth element. She expresses her earth element by grounding herself through special moments spent with family or friends, with an emphasis on eye contact, laughter, and physical embrace. She counters the moments of interaction with quiet periods with her Self.

Having moved through the process of harmonizing four of her inner elements, she easily phases into the expression of her metal element, which consists of doing at least one activity a day that stimulates her brain — maybe reading about a new topic, or doing the *New York Times* crossword puzzle (or just an easy online crossword puzzle). She also puts "happy brain" food in her body, like salmon and walnuts.

This harmonious mama makes a habit of living in a space of good vibes, even when the meconium is hitting the fan.

An Onslaught of Opinions

Ignorance was not bliss during my first trimester. I had no clue how I wanted to grow, birth, or nurture a baby — my feng shui was way off. I was met with many opinions laced with judgment, but few people advised me to follow my own instincts and do what *I* felt was right. I was told to get an epidural because "why not," or have a natural home birth because hospitals were "medicalized, corporate monsters." There seemed to be no loving middle ground.

I quickly discovered that childbirth opinions were often shared with an attitude: "There is my way or the wrong way, and no in between." My morning sickness was replaced by a nauseating sense that *someone* would be rolling their eyes at me regardless of the choices I made. I became so disheartened by the unsolicited advice I got (primarily from strangers) that I learned to discern what "team" each person was playing on and to mold my responses to placate their biases. I was unconsciously playing into the competitive nature of birth, and it did not feel authentic or nurturing. I let my pregnancy be about everyone but me — until I stopped.

The Birthing Divide

Roller Derby girls have nothing on the competing Childbirth Teams. On one side are the proponents of medical-free home births, on the other, the women who preorder their cocktail of birthing drugs before their first ultrasound. Caught in the crosshairs of this catfight are untold women who are not yet sure what they want but are hesitant to ask questions and fearful of being judged. This book is the voice of the middle ground, and the referee, me, is kindly asking everyone to take a time-out.

The competitive birthing culture isn't allowed in this space. Here, there are no teams to choose from. *Feng Shui Mommy* is an oasis that welcomes all, encouraging each woman to unapologetically embrace her own journey. This book gives you permission to follow your own path to birth and beyond.

My goal is to help you feel optimally equipped for *your* pregnancy and birth — not mine, not your mother's, not your doctor's, and certainly not your nosy Pilates instructor's. My job is to help you step out of the muck of expectation and cultural pressure so you can decide for yourself how you want to experience this life-altering adventure. The only people you need to listen to are yourself and your baby; the rest is, as they say, just noise. This is your time to hold the maternity and motherhood talking stick everyone else has been hogging.

Energized Curiosity

Growing a human is fascinating work. The science and spirituality entwined in the process are spectacular. While you read this book, you'll be galvanized to ask questions, examine the many sides of each answer, and choose the plan that is unique to you. So create time and space to allow this to happen.

Finding Your Tribe

Although you have everything you need between the top of your head and the tips of your toes to experience a wonderful birth, it doesn't hurt to have additional minds, hearts, and hands — preferably hands that don't mind pitching in and doing some cooking and cleaning, or offering to come over to hold the baby while you "de-gunk." Gathering your baby-raising villagers is an integral component of this journey.

Pregnancy and early motherhood can be drenched in feelings of isolation if you don't actively invite the right people into your experience. Pregnant women too often live in a state of quiet shame, certain that their fears, needs, and questions are too silly to share. But there are no silly questions when it comes to birthing; you are, after all, creating a whole new person.

Your journey should be one of mutual support, compassion, and unity. When you open yourself to the realization that you do not need to do this alone, and shouldn't do it alone, you will ease into a state of security where you feel free to express your vulnerability, and to request and accept help. From this space of security and vulnerability you will discover who will best support you during pregnancy and childbirth, and who will be generous with their heart and outstretched arms in the first chapters of your new life with your baby.

Your Map

Feng Shui Mommy is organized in four sections — First Trimester, Second Trimester, Third Trimester, and Fourth Trimester — with each section containing Mind, Body, and Spirit subsections.

Each chapter begins with a simple breathing exercise, allowing you to clear your mind and release any stress you may be holding so you can enjoy and absorb what you're reading. At the end of every chapter, you will find a simple riddle. The answer will be the offer code for a relaxation recording download created for that chapter, which you will be given the link to. These recordings will ensure that the insights you received while reading the book can be fully integrated into your subconscious mind, and they will give you a peaceful place to visit whenever you feel you've let some prenatal stress wiggle its way in. Following each riddle, you'll find a Call to Pleasure checklist of clear action steps you can take to infuse the Feng Shui Mommy harmony into your life.

Throughout the first trimester, *Feng Shui Mommy* leads you through the process of balancing the energies of your mind and physical surroundings, developing healthy practices to best nurture your body, and opening your spirit to the possibility of replacing your fears with courage. The Mind section resets your beliefs about the journey to motherhood and offers tangible and metaphysical resources to enrich your physical environments with nourishing energy. The Body section delivers an easy-to-navigate exercise and nutrition guide, geared to support you in achieving vibrant health during and after pregnancy — and it even gives you permission to eat some chocolate (not that you need permission). The Spirit section allows you to root out fears that are preventing you from fully enjoying the discoveries you will make on this new path. With the guidance of *Feng Shui Mommy*, you will come to the end of your first trimester with a sense of empowerment and positive anticipation.

As you step into your second trimester, *Feng Shui Mommy* supports you through the surge of events, planning, physical and spiritual changes, and needed resources that arrive with this "Golden Age" of pregnancy. In the Mind section, you will find the needed lens to view with calm and clarity events like the restructuring of your bedroom and the creation of your birth preferences. The Body section opens you to the sacred gifts of water and stokes your confidence in the face of any potential complications — setting the stage for your optimal birth. In the Spirit section, *Feng Shui Mommy* teaches you to access your inner sanctuary using self-hypnosis techniques. As you transition out of this midsection of your pregnancy, you will feel encouraged about your ability to transform your motherhood dreams into a juicy new reality.

Feng Shui Mommy's guidance during the final stage of pregnancy will flood you with a sense of excitement and flush away your fears of the unknown. The Mind section offers simple advice for creating your birthing sanctuary, ensuring that you feel nourished on your big day. In the Body section, the mysteries of the phases of birth are unveiled, and a light is shone on the physical positions and techniques you can use to remain strong, yet relaxed and comfortable, during the birth experience (and yes, there will be squatting). In the Spirit section, focus is placed on your breath, and unearthing the potential for pain relief and spiritual connection that live in it. You will end the third trimester thriving with a sense of accomplishment and unfathomable love for your Self and your new baby. *Yes! You will have a baby!*

Feng Shui Mommy honors and acknowledges the fourth trimester — the first few months of motherhood. The Mind chapter includes tips on how to stay connected to and nurture your new Self. The Body section offers insight into the gift of breastfeeding, postpartum surprises your body may encounter (hello, maxi pads!), and the basic, yet often surprising bodily functions of your baby (hello, diaper blowouts!). The Spirit passage will discuss how to deepen the connection between yourself and your new baby.

From Her Heart to Yours

Throughout the book I share the wisdom of women who candidly discuss the questions, confusions, and bursts of euphoria they experienced on their journey to motherhood. These morsels of wisdom and honesty are meant to connect you with the energy of other mothers, serving to lift you out of the sense of loneliness that can color pregnancy. The purpose of these stories is to expand your community of support and fill your heart with the power of sisterhood.

RIDDLE: I am the organ that will be your baby's safe haven until birth. What's my name?

Go to **YourSereneLife.wordpress.com/intro** and use the one-word riddle answer as your offer code to download the relaxation recording for this chapter. (It will make the one-dollar download free!)

CALL TO PLEASURE

- Spend five minutes, every day, visualizing your ideal birth.
- If in doubt, take a deep breath (and listen to the relaxation recording download).
- List all your pregnancy- and birthing-related questions, and make sure to include those you find weird. No need to find answers yet, just questions.
- Using the following questions as your guide, begin making a list of your tribe members:
  - Who will best support my needs during pregnancy?
  - Who will nurture my transition through birth?
  - Who will be generous with support in the first chapters of my new life with Baby?

FIRST TRIMESTER

A TIME
of
TRANSFORMATION

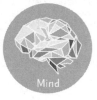

CHAPTER ONE

RECLAIMING SERENITY

JUST BREATHE: *Focus your attention on your breath. Envision peace, clarity, and courage flowing in with each inhalation, while fear, tension, and stress flow out with every exhalation. You emit a brightening glow with each breath, until you find yourself enveloped in healing energy. Let this energy enter every nerve and cell of your being — centering you for your reading experience.*

The most zealous of all the sperm has nuzzled into your waiting egg, and it's all systems go. Your body (and mind, and spirit) are now pooling their reserves of building blocks to create a new human. How do you feel about that? Thrilled? Terrified? In denial? Whatever your answer is, it is perfect. Pregnancy is the epitome of change, and it's your prerogative to completely freak out (in a good or bad way) over this development. It's strange to have a brand-new person growing inside of you! It's extraordinary! It is an everyday miracle in a global sense, but a cataclysmic shift in a personal sense. You are allowed to break down, whatever that looks like for you. There's no time when it's more socially acceptable to "lose it" than when you find out you're pregnant. And by losing it, you just might find all of it.

Pregnancy can trigger an identity crisis. You are no longer the person you thought you were, but you are not yet the person you will become. It's a time of awesome transition and change, which is always scary. Becoming a mother doesn't mean you stop being yourself — your fun Self, your carefree Self, your sensual Self. What it does mean is that you have the unique opportunity to become the person you truly want to be, the person you're meant to be: a woman who experiences herself as centered, whole, and stronger than she's ever been before, your true Self. During this time, your feng shui, composed of the energy connecting your mind, body, and spirit, is shaken up in the great cosmic maternal martini shaker — and you don't even get to have a drink! But once the head spinning slows, you will find that you have more resources, more resilience, and more creativity than ever before.

It's All Connected

Because you are a holistic being, your mind, body, and spirit are designed to work together in a state of dynamic fluidity, constantly realigning around your optimal balance point. When you bring awareness to this connectivity, you allow powerful change to happen.

Pregnancy is a profound chapter of life, for sure, but it's not the whole story. What pregnancy offers is a chance to get your holistic house in order so you are beautifully prepared for the rest of your life. Now is the time to find your joyful and courageous core. Now is the time to connect with your authentic and best Self.

Eating fried bacon–wrapped pastries for breakfast but thinking happy thoughts won't optimize your holistic connection. Doing an hour of yoga while focusing on the stressful tasks you have to do afterward won't optimize your holistic connection. Removing your partner's action figure collection from the bedroom while panicking about your future ability to breastfeed won't optimize your holistic connection. What will optimize it is becoming grounded in your experience, learning to express your needs, and finding the right kind of support.

Releasing the Fear

"The agony of childbirth" is one of the most pervasive messages in our culture. The first image of birth I was exposed to was a sweaty, red-faced woman, screaming PG-13-rated profanities at her partner while nudging a human out of her vagina in a comical movie. It was hilarious, and horrifying. I've never seen one scripted birthing image in the media that doesn't contain terrified men, yelling — and needles, so many needles! The births that are featured on reality shows are often flush with trauma and "excitement." Anxious voices, screaming, and tears sell, I guess. Peaceful companions, gentle births, and intact perinea are "boring."

The frightful cousins of these traumatic birth images are the harrowing sagas many women relish sharing about their excruciating forty-hour births, emergency C-sections, and bruised babies being yanked from tiny vaginas. Our society is a cultivator of childbirthing fear. Fear that we'll grow a child who is not brimming with health. Fear that our bodies will forget how to birth when the time comes. Fear that we'll make a critical mistake and dismantle our optimal birth.

This fear can turn a self-assured, courageous, and intelligent woman into a quivering mess. In addition to the external bombardment of fear, that little bratty voice within, the inner critic, loves to repeatedly ask, "*How the hell is that going to squeeze out of this tiny hole?*" Knowing that countless other women have accomplished this feat helps a bit, but the thought still lingers that those other vaginas were somehow...better at this.

There is another way. There is a healing room within you that holds space for the opposite of fear — hope, courage, and empowerment. These forces are much stronger than fear; they just need some encouragement from you to come forth. When fear of childbirth is exposed to the light of reality, it begins to fade. This opens the door of possibility for your experience to be flush with joy, relaxation, and happiness. And fun! Believe it or not, pregnancy, childbirth, and motherhood can actually be fun.

In the end, when I got over the initial terror of it all, I had a really fun pregnancy. But I did not wake up one morning with a sudden gusto for this process. I had to do heaps of fear-release work before I felt at ease with the prospect of a big head with a long body attached coming out of my body. So I invite you to meditate on the notion that when you release the fear, the possibilities will rush in (we'll dig into this further in chapter 6).

Wisdom to Remember

Long ago, in a land far away, fear did not grip the guts of pregnant women. In ancient times, childbirth was viewed as an organic, orgasmic process, as natural as a bowel movement, albeit a sacred one. The birthing stories that were passed from woman to woman possessed a tone of spirituality, connection, and knowing. Women trusted that their bodies were made for childbirth and that their babies would cooperate in the process. Birthing women and birth keepers in these times were revered as goddesses, able to channel the sacred creation of new life. So what the hell happened?

The reverence ended when pregnant women who needed medical assistance began to be viewed by law as "undeserving ill." The gross logic went like this: these women must have committed some kind of "sin," otherwise their pregnancies would not be complicated. Then the real craziness kicked in: Doctors were forbidden to offer care to these women, and as a result many died. These unnecessary tragedies planted in pregnant women the seed of fear that they too would be denied medical care if they needed it. This was the dawning of the culture of fear that still surrounds childbirth today. While this fear is still a powerful force, it has no basis in reality.

The medical resources of the modern healthcare system have significantly improved, and, compared with the era when this "culture of fear" arose, today it is much rarer for a woman in need of these resources to not receive them. But that old fear persists, and it has colored how many in the medical profession (and the media) still view women and childbirth.

It's time to put this fear down for a permanent nap.

Spiritual Intention and Introspection

Women used to place as much focus on the spiritual intentions of their pregnancy as we now place on combing through baby-stuff reviews. Navajos honored the divine feminine power of the pregnant woman with a ceremony called a Blessingway, which inspired what many now call a Mother's Blessing. This Blessingway celebrated the woman's rite of passage into her new identity as a mother, and set the intention that with the growth of the baby came the growth of the mother's spirit.

In "Navajo Ceremonial System," Leland C. Wyman explains that

"Blessingway is concerned with peace, harmony, and good things exclusively … for good hope, for good luck, to avert misfortune, to invoke positive blessings.… Thus they [Blessingways] are used to aid childbirth." Blessingway ceremonies, which would often span "from sundown of one day to dawn of the second day after that," often consisted of chanting and prayer, and as Wyman explains, "there is a ritual bath in the forenoon, sometimes drypaintings made of variously colored cornmeal, pulverized flower petals, and pollens strewn on a buckskin or a cloth substitute spread on the ground, with more songs and prayers. The final night is taken up with all-night singing."

You may not be up for a forty-eight-ish-hour ceremony. But your spiritual life is important right now. When you purposefully pay homage to the miracle of pregnancy, you take back your power. You no longer feel like a victim of circumstance, especially if your pregnancy was unplanned, like my own was. Set the intention that the being who is meant to come to you will, and trust that your baby is choosing you for a reason. Cultivating this trust can be especially beneficial for parents of children who come into this world with special needs.

Instead of focusing on your identity as changing, think of it as expanding. As your belly grows, so does your place in the world.

From Her Heart to Yours

I once heard a spiritual leader say that nine months of pregnancy, if harnessed in its potential power and ability to heal, is equivalent to twenty years of meditation. I realized that my unborn child was presenting me with a chance to look at, resolve, understand, repattern, and mend things that perhaps never would have emerged had I not become pregnant with her. Like an angel, it appeared that this was in fact one of the purposes of her coming into the world, to assist me in healing pieces of myself, my history and my ancestry, that would affect not only me — but how she, herself, experienced life. Within me arose this primal urge to give her the best possible future, free of the things that weighed me down. I didn't want to pass them on to her. I wanted the buck to stop here. I wanted to gift her a legacy of healing, not of wounds. One of courage and strength. One of love, compassion, optimism, and hope; power, truth, and grace.

— *Jessica Cauffiel, California*
(mom, actor, writer, producer, shaman, and spiritual rockstar)

Magnifying Intuition

Intuition used to be queen. Women valued the voice of their intuition above all else — more than the voice of their mother, their sister, their guru, their cat, and (gasp) even their doctor. A woman's intuition led the journey, plotted new trails, and drew the map.

The first of the three elements of faith in Buddhism is intuition. Listening to this "gut reaction" or "sixth sense" is the first door that must be opened in order to access the other two core elements of Buddhist faith, which are reason and experience. When birthing, Tibetan Buddhists are encouraged to follow the wisdom of their subconscious, turning inward to discover right action. Our intuitions, however, have been shoved into the dark recesses of our psyches and rarely see the light of our consciousness. But tapping into your intuition — by listening to the first voice that answers in the moment after we ask our Self a question, before the mental chatter begins — is crucial to a successful birth, so we must learn to trust and follow that sacred inner voice. When we unlock this voice of wisdom, the important questions we're being asked, or are asking, will be answered.

Tapping Into Your Creativity

I remember oozing with pride, and a little cockiness, when, as an eleven-year-old hiking in the mountains of West Texas, I discovered a little cave whose walls were covered in petroglyphs. These ancient drawings depicted new life: seeds transforming into thriving trees, buds unfolding into blossoms, and a voluptuous stick figure depositing humans from her womb. It was a wonderfully scandalous discovery for a prepubescent girl. I envisioned glowing Native American pregnant women floating into the cave, their hands drawing on the cool rock.

For too many of us, fear has stifled our creative expression. Instead of working through the flux of emotions that pregnancy brings by tapping into our creativity, we use television, sleep, or my personal favorite, sweets, to check out when the new and potentially uncomfortable emotions check in. While the treats of entertainment, rest, and food are wonderful, they don't facilitate the exploration of the physical, emotional, and spiritual changes of pregnancy.

When you feel overcome by the unknown, follow the lead of our ancient Native American sisters and utilize a creative medium of your choosing to explore the questions, insights, or bursts of transformation you are experiencing.

If you feel separated from your changing body, turn on some music and dance. Allow movement to reconnect your body with your spirit, so you feel at home in your morphing body. If you have dreams you would like to consciously explore, paint your impressions of these visions on canvas. If you have powerful emotions surrounding a relationship, use free-flow writing to allow the voice of your intuition to speak up. Much like the act of putting on your shoes to exercise, the hardest part is turning on the music, picking up the paintbrush, or opening the journal. The rest is magic.

And if you, like me, just end up drawing pregnant stick figures — that's great too!

Uplifting Storytelling

Our foremothers spoke of the grace, wisdom, and expansion of childbirth. Their stories were not laced with warnings and trauma, but neither did they deny the reality that childbirth is a challenge. The purpose of the stories was not for personal aggrandizement, but to uplift and encourage their sisters who were stepping into their own experience. These women wanted their sisters to reach the great moment of release — birth — filled with hope and expectation, and a sense of awe.

In ancient Malaysia and Indonesia, mothers would surround a birthing woman and offer to tell the tales of their own births. If the laboring woman moved into a challenge during birth, a supportive sister would share words of hope and insight from a similar experience. These tales served to instill a belief in the woman in transition that she was protected by the women who had traveled this path before her.

Feng Shui Mommy is a call to action to speak our birth stories with reverence, positivity, and truth. Our C-sections, epidurals, natural births, squatting births, and belly-dancing births — all are as valuable as the next in this space.

So set the intention that you will attract positive birth stories. Ask the women in your tribe to share positive childbirth stories with you, or find women who can. Find a special time and place to gather these women and fill the space with the electric energy of encouragement. Record these stories, or take notes, so you can draw from this optimistic wisdom anytime you need a dose of "Yes I can." Tell anyone who lapses into framing their birthing story as a calamity that you will only listen to her tale of woe if she is willing to rub your feet while she's telling it.

Prenatal Bonding

Tibetans have long held the belief that you must fill your baby with love before she is born, ensuring she enters this strange new world with deep reserves of assurance and comfort, which will soothe and support her when she is feeling out of sorts.

A baby in utero can hear the melody of your voice, feel the intention in your touch, and taste the flavors of the foods you eat. Prenatal care and bonding used to be viewed as a sacred time that warranted just as much attention as the first few weeks of the newborn's life. This prebirth bonding period served to gradually connect the mother and baby well before they came face to face.

It can be difficult to absorb how a new human will fit into your life. You've settled into your patterns, social groups, and the diaper-less landscape of your life. The idea of bringing a new human, completely dependent on you, into this scene is daunting.

When I first felt my baby move, I sat on my bed in an absolute state of awe. There was a person inside of me! This person was going to come out of me, and this person would be in my life forever. I tried to conjure images of what this child would look like, hoping he would be a bit plumper than the darling scrawny figure on the ultrasound printouts. I tried to imagine what it would feel like to have this child try to obtain milk from my tiny breasts — What if he didn't get enough food? What if he didn't thrive? Wait a minute — Who was I to take care of a baby?...and before I knew it, my moment of bliss had become obliterated by fear and doubt. I realized then that looking too far ahead wasn't good for me. Instead, I had to circle back and find my way into the peace of the present moment.

I stopped jumping forward, and focused instead on connecting with the baby who was inside of me. I talked to him, I sang to him, I danced with him, I asked him what he felt like eating (frozen yogurt), I wrote to him, I read to him (mystery romance thrillers), and generally included him in everything, except when I was having fantastic prenatal sex with his dad.

I bonded with my baby before I met him so I wouldn't feel like I was pushing a stranger out of my uterus when the time came.

Connect with your baby *now*. It doesn't matter if you're five weeks pregnant, five months pregnant, or even setting the intention that you will become pregnant. Make the connection now. Take quiet moments throughout your day to send love to your baby, and fill your days with nourishing your own body, mind, and soul, knowing you are also nourishing his.

Ritual

Tibetans believe that the spirit of their culture is passed through the rituals of childbirth. They partake in these rituals to ensure their heritage is passed from generation to generation. They chant affirmations, burn incense, beat cymbals and drums, and receive the blessings of monks. There is an auspicious nature to these rituals, serving to enhance the belief that women have a heightened connection to the spiritual realm during pregnancy. Mothers-to-be believe these ceremonies connect them with a higher power.

American culture lacks this type of ritual, but it doesn't have to. Affirmations, chanting, tokens of love, aromatic scents, sensual textures, purposeful eye contact, soul-soothing music, and other actions and symbols that hold a tone of blessing will serve to deepen your experience and move you into a space of appreciation and reverence for the new life you are creating.

Create your own rituals. Find a special hiking trail that calls to you, and walk it as the sun sets every Sunday evening. Continue this ritual after your child is born. Rise before the sun and sit with a hot cup of tea on a special chair as you greet the day. When your baby has entered this world, hold her in this chair and watch the sun rise with her. Creating rituals will add richness to your journey and take the edge off daily stressors.

I was naturally drawn to the ritual of staying in or around the house for the first forty days of my child's life. We kept the shades drawn and cocooned ourselves indoors, partially because the brutal summer heat of Ojai, California, was unforgiving. This ritual was lovely and allowed me time to bond with Hudson before attempting to integrate both of us into the larger world beyond our home. The only time Eric and I broke this ritual was to take Hudson to a beach concert in Santa Monica and... *What were we thinking?* We both learned that it's important to respect the ritual.

Trusting the Body

The female body was created to birth new life. Ancient women knew this, respected this, and went with it. Ancient Egyptian women honored their bodies and the giver of life, the Great Mother, by belly dancing. They believed belly dancing heightened the body's ability to create — especially to create another being. Belly dancing was used before conception to attract the new life, during pregnancy to strengthen the abdominal muscles, and throughout birth to spiral the energetic force of gravity down and out. These gyrations allowed the woman to trust in and surrender to the natural forces of her body. Many of us have lost this trust in our bodies and must rediscover and claim it by tuning in to the subtle messages of our bodies and allowing them to guide us.

The Cocoon of Support

Ancient art depicting childbirth often displays a group of attendants surrounding the birthing woman. Peter Paul Rubens's painting *The Birth of the Princess*, completed in the early 1570s, depicts the birth of a baby girl, the mother and child flanked by supporters and protectors. It used to be a given that the primary females in a woman's life would gather around her during birth.

Every woman deserves to have a supportive group of women in attendance at her birth. The challenge is to appropriately educate those around you so they play only a supportive and nurturing role, as opposed to demanding or distracting.

Create the intention that your ideal support group will come to you, meditate on who it might include, and be gentle with yourself when you realize that all the individuals who will want to be in the group may not be a great fit for your needs. Your birthing experience should be a natural and harmonious gathering of people who love you — and each other.

Gravitational Positions

There is a stone carving in Egypt, in the Temple of Hathor at Dendera, that depicts a squatting woman being supported by two goddesses. This is not unusual; I have never seen ancient art depicting a woman lying flat on her back with her feet in stirrups.

It used to be understood that gravity is essential to the birthing process. Yet it has become common practice in hospitals for women to give birth lying flat on their back, feet up in metal stirrups, with a spotlight aimed at their vagina. This setup facilitates the care provider's comfort and ease — but not the mother's.

Getting friendly with gravity is a great thing to cultivate throughout your pregnancy. Notice how your body moves now that it is caring for another. How do your feet feel when they touch the ground? How does your seat feel when the earth supports it? Becoming attuned to yourself as a creature who roams the earth, and honoring yourself as this being, will better prepare you to follow your physical instincts when labor begins.

Animals Do It

The captivity of modern birthing culture has killed our animal birthing instincts. There is no better way to get back in touch with our primal instincts than to do what the animals do. Have you ever seen an animal give birth? They wait for the appropriate time, then let their bodies deposit their baby, without any fuss. It's instinctual, natural, and glorious. Because animals are deeply in tune with nature, they can sense when the time is right to relax, and when they will be safe. This means most animals give birth at night, under some kind of shelter, usually alone.

I know a woman who raises goats. These goats live *the life*. They reside on twenty acres of grassy, yodel-worthy meadows, and they pay rent with a bit of milk. One evening, Gertrude the goat started to show signs of labor. My goat-raising buddy led Gertrude into the barn. As labor progressed, a thunderstorm rolled in, and Gertrude promptly put her labor in a resting state; she sensed danger. As soon as nature's tantrum had ceased, Gertrude restarted her labor and her kid slid out. Animals are aligned with the energy of nature. They trust their bodies, and trust their environment. We humans need to remember to do this.

Throughout my pregnancy, I felt most at home outside. I knew that nature understood what I was going through. I would walk for hours, stopping to smell a flower, watch a few randy bees, or just lie in the grass and watch the clouds play. It was lovely and timeless. In these moments I was in a heightened state of awareness. I was in tune with my baby, my breath, and the blood pumping through me. I felt connected and soft, going back inside only when I got hungry.

During birth, I was stuck in a clinical hospital room, but I let my mind take me to a more serene place — the ocean. I visualized clean wave after wave surging, then crashing, then retreating as I labored.

Reconnecting to the knowing of animals and recognizing birth as one of the most natural acts in the universe released a great deal of fear in me, as it has done for the women I've worked with. Claim your right to a gentle, comfortable, and joyful state of being, then take another step in your epic journey to motherhood.

RIDDLE: What form of physical movement did ancient Egyptian women practice to attract new life? (Besides sex!)

Go to **YourSereneLife.wordpress.com/chapter-one** and use the two-word riddle answer as your offer code for the relaxation recording for this chapter.

CALL TO PLEASURE

- Find a token to symbolize your holistic unity (it can double as your birth token). Touch it whenever you need a reminder to tune back in to this unity.
- Hone your intuition by asking questions and then writing down the first answer that comes to you.
- Plan a female gathering to collect positive birth stories.
- Make up a weekly ritual that you will continue after your child is born.
- List your primary sources of fear. (Media? Certain friends?) Practice limiting your exposure to those sources.
- Tap into your creative medium of choice and spend one uninterrupted hour creating.

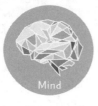

Mind

CHAPTER TWO

FENG SHUI
Harmonizing Your Outer and Inner Worlds

JUST BREATHE: *Allow your breath to deepen as you read this chapter, leading you into a space where you are acutely aware of how the energy surrounding you affects the energy within you — and how you can transform this energy to your liking.*

If you tune in to your emotions when you enter a space, you'll become aware of a shift in your energy. If the space has stagnant feng shui (a.k.a. "a stagnant flow of energy"), you'll experience a negative shift in energy. If the space has flowing feng shui, you'll experience a positive shift in energy.

You don't have control over many of the spaces you inhabit throughout your day, but you can enliven the energy in the spaces in your home. Because your home will be the main haven you and your energy-sensitive baby will reside in, you'll want it to be a positive-energy palace. Cultivating vibrant feng shui in your home will both soothe your baby and serve as your Cosmic Chill Pill. We concoct this chill pill by removing clutter and introducing air-purifying plants, fresh air, soothing lighting, and optimal colors into your home.

You don't need to be a compass-slinging wizard to receive the benefits of feng shui. Unifying the following ideas with your home and committing to daily "resetting" practices will organically begin the process of awakening your Goddess-Mama-Chi.

Organic Roommates

Nature dances with consciousness, which is why plants are feng shui masters; they exude positive energy without even trying. If you're starved for nature, or if you just like plants, incorporating house-plants (that *you* love) into your home will infuse it with grounding, cleansing, and nourishing energy. Plants also awaken the earth element, unifying you with whole-being nourishment, inner balance, and stability.

> P.S. *If you're nervous about taking care of a human, nurturing houseplants will be good practice — and you don't have to breast-feed them. (But you do need to speak baby-talk to them.)*

Because NASA is all about bringing people back to Earth, they conducted a study on the top air-purifying houseplants. Here are some plants you might find on the International Space Station, or in every room of my house.

- Peace lily (my go-to gal because she's pretty, and not too needy)
- Spider plant
- Bamboo palm
- Red-edged dracaena
- Florist's chrysanthemum
- English ivy

These plants remove toxic agents such as trichloroethylene, formaldehyde, benzene, and xylene from the air — toxins that create symptoms like dizziness; nausea; drowsiness and headache; an irritated mouth, nose, and throat; itchy eyes; elevated heart rate; heart issues; and liver and kidney damage. Yuck!

All these yummy chemicals are found in common household items like inks, varnishes, paper bags, wax paper, and more. And don't some of those symptoms sound like they were pulled from a "How to Know When You're Knocked Up" article? I wonder what pregnancy symptoms were like for women before the Industrial Revolution, when many people spent most of their days outdoors?

Because babies sometimes (always) enjoy putting *everything* in their

EXPERT TIP: *My thumb has more of a brown than green tinge, so I like to stick with plants that pretty much take care of themselves. Spider plants and peace lilies are my main tribe members. They forgive me my faults in the areas of soil health and water scheduling.*

mouths, ensure that the plants you're inviting in are displayed out of the reach of tiny hands, and the paws and teeth of the domesticated animal that may be following them.

Breathe in Fresh Energy

Tune in to your mind's nose and envision walking into a room filled with the lingering scent of stale cigarette smoke, mixed with a hint of dirty carpet and a whiff of forgotten garbage. How does that make you feel?

Now, clear your mind's nose and imagine walking into a space filled with fresh air, emanating with the aroma of freshly cut grass, a hint of jasmine, and an undertone of clean energy (whatever clean energy might smell like). When you breathe in this air, it feels crisp and invigorating, as if it's replenishing your body's reserve of fuel. Does that feel better?

The air you breathe translates into the energy you breathe. This energetic oxygen is absorbed by your baby, affecting how his developmental building blocks are pieced together. Gift yourself and your babe with clean air by opening windows when the weather is nice (placing a window guard in the window when your baby becomes mobile and curious) or utilizing one or many of the air-purifying plants previously listed. Small fountains are also pros at humidifying and refreshing air.

Make a ritual of opening the windows or caring for your plants. As you open the window, close your eyes and inhale deeply, imagining the fresh air resetting your system and connecting you to the present moment. Then, imagine it flowing into your baby and your home, clearing out negative energy and blessing everything (and everyone) it touches. When you open your eyes everything will look brighter and crisper.

If you're relying on vegetation to cleanse your air, say a blessing of gratitude to each plant as you feed it water or prune dead leaves. Plants have been found to positively respond to sound, so speak sweet somethings to them, or play them your favorite music while envisioning the good vibrations absorbing into their roots.

Clear That Clutter

Feng shui is in a love affair with simplicity. Overloading any space you inhabit (your home, your mind, your body, your spirit, your time, etc.) pulls you down and can make even the smallest task as crushing as a steamroller. Clearing, cleaning, and lightening the spaces you inhabit frees you from heavy energy, lifting you above any tendencies toward the tedious.

Clutter is confusing — it confuses the energy in our outer environment, which translates into a chaotic inner environment. I cannot think of anything productive when I'm sitting in clutter. Before I became a good-natured tyrant toward my stuff, I used to work in my car because it was the only place I could concentrate. There were entire rooms in my home that served as junk drawers, and they made me feel really heavy. I've had to help many organizing clients (and myself) escape the catch-22 of organizing: multiple "heavy" spaces make you feel chained to your home because you feel like you need to do something about them, but because you feel so heavy you have little motivation, or clarity of thought, to make any progress. Ugh. Damn you, junk rooms!

Move past this catch-22 by focusing on the simple mantra, "If it doesn't add immense happiness or value to my life, I will let it go." Then go through your home and throw away or donate anything that doesn't sync with that maxim. One (wo)man's old good-energy-sucking television set is another (wo)man's box of treasures that will be used for an art project, so it is unfair of you to keep items that add no positivity to your life, but that could be a total score in someone else's. Free your Self by freeing your stuff.

> ADDED BONUS: *A clutter-free home equals less random stuff for Baby to put in her mouth. So while you're decluttering, you're also babyproofing.*

I have a vision of you walking through your spaces and feeling joy or appreciation for everything you look at — nothing is weighing you down, and everything has a home. I love that.

Soothing Lighting

Serenity emanates from positive lighting, and it's drained away by negative lighting. Because light is one of the strongest sources of energy, its intentional use is a crucial ingredient for the nest of love you're creating for your sprout.

Let's first eliminate the positive-energy-killing vortex of fluorescent lighting. Fluorescent lights — yuck! Have you ever thought, "Dang, I look sexy!" when trying on a bikini standing in a dressing room under a buzzing light that accentuates every rivet of cellulite? Fluorescent light is draining and makes everything look like a pasty version of itself. I no longer say, "I'm in a bad mood" — I say, "I'm in a fluorescent lighting mood" (spiritually pasty, mentally cranky, and physically cellulite-y). This type of lighting is so bad it has been banned in Germany. So permanently turn off your fluorescent lights, or swap them out for ambient lighting, if possible.

> MAMA TIP: *If your baby experiences jaundice (a common medical condition with yellowing of the skin or the whites of the eyes), your pediatrician will likely recommend exposing him to natural light.*

So now that you've smashed your fluorescent lights...fill the darkness with soft, warm, and well-placed lighting. Natural light is queen during the day, so open up your blinds and let the good vibes (and vitamin D!) flow in.

In the evenings, I love lamps. I love them so much I've lit many of my bathrooms with lamps, rather than vanity lighting. I don't put my makeup on as well, but dang, that soft lighting makes me *think* I look good! When the sun is sleeping, turn on at least three sources of light at three different levels in the room you're occupying. In many of my rooms I have one or two floor lamps, and two tabletop lamps. In more intimate areas, like your bedroom or nursery, limit the use of overhead lighting. And because babies and cords are often equivalent to cats and yarn, make sure all cords are out of Baby's reach.

From Her Heart to Yours

When my husband turned on the overhead light in our bedroom every morning, it was my trigger to get up and throw up during my pregnancy. My room would go from a dark and gentle haven to a stark and bland box. I really disliked that light. To soothe my belly, I would leave my room, grab a glass of water, and sit in a rocking chair in my living room, which was coated in natural light. The deeper I swam into pregnancy, the more I tuned in to how my five (sometimes six) senses were connected to my mental, physical, and spiritual well-being. An "aha lightbulb" (hehe) flipped on one morning as my husband turned on The Light. I asked him to switch it off and open the blinds instead. The moment the harsh light was replaced by nature's gentle glow, my stomach settled and vomiting ceased to be part of my morning ritual. I am now lulled awake by Mother Nature, not the flickering from a manmade tube.

— J. K., Austin, Texas

Optimal Colors

Colors emit messages that are absorbed by the eyes, perceived in the mind, and felt in the soul. The colors surrounding you should be harmonious with the needs within you. Particular characteristics emanate from different hues, making them prime influencers of your inner climate. It's like each color is a guru for different emotions.

But you're the Master Guru of your emotions, so follow your intuition when introducing new colors into your home. If the color *feels* good to you, you're exploring the right part of the rainbow. If a color you introduce into a space feels off, kick it out.

> **SOLACE FOR YOUR SANITY**: *Because babies are mega-channels of the energy around them, it's in your favor to keep the colors in the primary spaces Baby will occupy soft and soothing. Think gentle earth tones, or Easter-pastel chic.*

A Guide to Your Emotion Gurus

Yellow

The golden guru of inner warmth, hope, and miracles. You can soak in the warming effects of yellow during all waking hours by indirectly gazing into the glint of the sun, the glow of a lamp, or a favorite item or image that is kissed by yellow. If you feel yourself sinking into a funk, seek out something in a shade of yellow, focusing on the hue until you become aware that your spirits are being brightened.

Orange

The guru of success, fresh life, and renewal. Orange radiates zesty fun, pulling you out of the monotonous by sparking fresh ideas and enthusiasm for creating powerful shifts in your life. Hold something orange when you need an extra dose of inspiration.

Red

The guru of sexual energy and the invigorator of romance, courage, and adventure. Red evokes vitality and passion, serving to enliven your physicality if you're feeling romantically dry, bodily drained, or internally depleted. Hang an image that's heavy with the tone of red in your bedroom to focus on when your libido needs incentive to get going.

Pink

The guru of nourishment and creativity. Pink ignites whimsy and imagination, guiding you into a dreamy, contemplative space where you can play with ideas without being weighed down by their potential pitfalls. Place a pink Himalayan salt crystal lamp in the bedroom or nursery to invite in a nurturing presence.

Purple

The guru of grace, honor, and exploration. Purple inspires the spirit to dive into its past, unearthing forgotten "knowings" and wisdom. This regal color supports you in realizing your highest ideals, which can serve as your beacon of intention. This is a helpful color to have near when you're creating your birth preferences.

Blue

The guru of fluid serenity. Blue demands nothing of you, allowing you to just *be*. Blue is a wonderful color to lean into when life seems chaotic and overwhelming, because it leads you back to your loving center and inspires a deep trust for the voice of your intuition. Because of its calming nature, blue was my "birth color" (the color I focused on during birth), and it's the birth color of many of my clients.

Green

The guru of health and renewal. Green is a direct link to the natural world and the wisdom of Mother Nature. Green helps to harmonize your heart energy with your emotions, supporting you in times of transformation and rebirth. This color can be good inspiration if you need to make big decisions or begin big projects.

Light Brown/Beige

The guru of simplicity. I'd like to reframe the common misconception of beige as boring or bland so that it's recognized as an enhancer of clarity and calm. Beige is a favorite feng shui color for nursery rooms as it promotes nourishment, inner balance, stability, and health — good stuff for Mom and Babe.

Because the emotions of the other people living in your home matter, have them weigh in on how the colors you're introducing make them feel. You don't want to be the only blissed-out babe in the house.

> RIDDLE: What is the destroyer of positive energy, now banned in Germany?
>
> Go to **YourSereneLife.wordpress.com/chapter-two** and use the two-word riddle answer as your offer code to download the relaxation recording for this chapter.

CALL TO PLEASURE

- Choose one or two of your favorite air-purifying plants and place one in each of the primary rooms where you and Baby will spend time (and put them in colorful pots that make you *feel* good!).
- On warm days, make a ritual of opening up your windows every

morning, closing your eyes, and feeling the fresh air move in and out of your nostrils.

- Clutter — clear it! Keep a donation box in an out-of-the-way, but convenient, location and place one unneeded item in it daily.
- Inspire good energy in every room by placing three sources of warm (nonfluorescent!) lighting at three different levels.
- Fill your home with colors that make you feel amazing. Paint the walls, display your *favorite* pieces of colorful art or keepsakes, or find throw pillows in colors that make you smile.
- Keep your chi flowing by keeping your home and mind clutter free (hello donation boxes, to-do lists, and journals!), committing to nourishing your physical and spiritual needs daily, making the exploration of your creativity a priority, spending quality time with your loved ones and your Self, and keeping your mind sharp with brain games (or anything else that makes you furrow your brow).

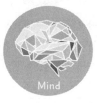

CHAPTER THREE

NONTRADITIONAL HEALING THROUGH EFT AND SHAKING

Just Breathe: *Set the intention that the deep breathing you will engage in while you read this chapter (breathing in for eight counts, holding for two, out for eight) will train your lungs to always follow this slow and steady pattern — even when your mind is trying to stress you out.*

Did you know that tapping on points in various regions of your head and upper body, and encouraging your body to shake, could change your life? Did you know this tapping and shaking could be your safe channel to release fears of flying, urges to scream profanities at careless drivers, chronic pain, proclivities for instant cake mixes, fear of infant poop, or anything else you no longer want stuck to your psyche? (Oh yeah, and childbirth — these exercises help you release resistance to childbirth.)

Just Tap It Out: Emotional Freedom Technique (EFT)

An electrical system runs through your body, humming with the power to shift negative emotions, trauma, fears, jealousy, stress, fatigue, nausea, and other inhabitants of the shadows into rainbow-hued flecks of light (like hope, release, giggles, acceptance, peace, and other brands of sunshine) — when it's working properly.

This system is temperamental, and when in disarray it causes us to feel like a metaphorical television set with a screwdriver jammed into the wires. And then pregnancy comes along, one-ups the screwdriver, and kicks the television set off a cliff. Emotional Freedom Technique (EFT) was created to piece that TV back together, pull out the screwdriver, and reset those wires, allowing our screen to hum with vibrant life and color.

This energy, or chi, we're working with runs through pathways called *meridians* (the same pathways used in acupuncture and acupressure). The existence of this energy is not hypothetical — it is measured and monitored by medical professionals via EEGs and EKGs, devices that measure the electrical activity in the brain and heart.

A poor diet, joy, stress, injury, a juice cleanse, disease, excitement, pregnancy — *anything and everything* impacts our electrical system, yet it is often the forgotten child who sulks in the corner. When that child is in distress or feeling neglected, it's really difficult to get him to do anything positive. To harmonize the energy (and cheer up that kid!) through EFT, we tap with our fingers on the end points of the body's energy meridians while meditating on the problem we want to resolve. The charge of the energy, for that particular issue, shifts from negative to positive.

Occasionally, wires get crossed, and the negative energy created from, say, a social anxiety could manifest in chronic pain in the lower back. Soothing the energy of the social anxiety could provide the secondary benefit of releasing the back pain.

To start, I'll need you to buy some witch hazel, red yarn, a dream catcher, and an extendable back scratcher....

Just kidding. Do you have your mind and fingers on deck? Perfect. Let's begin tapping it out.

Setup: Level of Distress and Affirmation

Before you begin resetting your energy around a particular issue, you need to decide what issue you would like to work with. For example, the first time I tapped, I focused on my panic-attack-inducing fear of flying. Once you clear the energy for one issue, you can move on to others.

Because this book is about your journey into motherhood, we'll use "fear of childbirth" as our example. We first need to determine how much distress this issue is causing you. Close your eyes and focus on your fear of childbirth. Decide what your current level of distress is on a scale of zero to ten — zero being no pain or anxiety around childbirth, and ten being extreme pain or anxiety around childbirth.

Next, we need to tune your energy system in to the issue we'll be working on. To do this, locate two tender spots about two or three inches below your collarbone on each side of your chest. Rub those spots in a circular motion while saying the following affirmation three times out loud (or in your head):

"Although I have a fear of childbirth, I still profoundly and wholly love and honor myself." (Again, say this while rubbing your upper chest, not your boobs.)

You can do this for any issue: just say "Although I have a [insert issue here], I still profoundly and wholly love and honor myself." So if you want to do this for a specific discomfort during childbirth, you could say, "Although I have pressure and pulling in my lower back, I still profoundly and wholly love and honor myself."

Tapping Points

Your energetic fear of childbirth (or spiders, or reality television, or fill in the blank) is now ripe for the resetting. Following the numbers on the diagram on the next page, tap each point while repeating your affirmation. Use your pointer finger and middle finger on each hand, so you can cover each side of your body simultaneously with each round.

In other words, you'll tap point 1, at the inner corner of your eyebrow, six to eight times while saying the affirmation once. Then on to point 2. You'll say the affirmation ten times in all, once at each tapping point.

Repeat the sequence a few times, then close your eyes and sit in silence for a few moments.

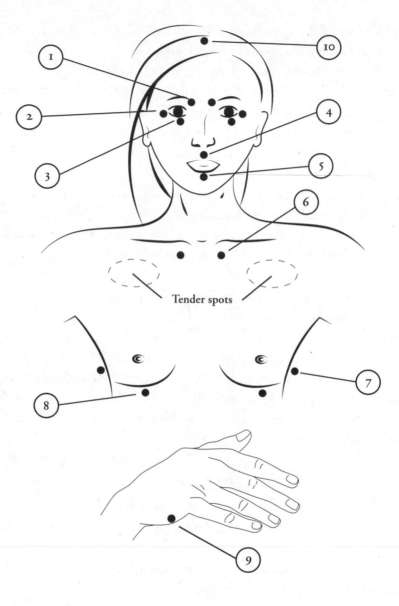

Tender spots

Reassessment

As you sit with yourself, reassess your level of distress over the issue you're working with. Using our baby-birthing example, imagine you're deep in childbirth. See and *feel* yourself there, noticing what comes up. You may still experience hints of fear or anxiety, but likely not at the same level as before you tapped your energetic meridians.

You now go through a few more rounds of the tapping sequence, this time using a revised affirmation:

"Although I still have *some* fear of childbirth, I still profoundly and wholly love and honor myself."

We're still acknowledging the fear, but honoring the reduction of its intensity.

Continue the cycle of tapping, affirmations, and reassessment until your intensity level is down to a zero (or whatever number you feel good with). I just took a break from typing to tap out my anxiety over the one-week colon cleanse I'm about to start. Cayenne pepper and warm lemon water is no joke.

Turn Your Goo into Wings:
Why You Should Encourage Your Body to Shake

Did you know that when you're heart-deep in an intense situation (one that the mind often labels as "bad") and you begin shaking and feeling like you're buzzing, you're actually moving through a metamorphosis? What, you're already doing it? Hey, Girl, you're turning into a butterfly! But wait — you didn't transform completely? Why not? Did you resist the shaking? Did you make it stop? Did you shut it down before your wings could grow?

Allowing your body to shake when you're moving through a tense situation is like weeding out all levels of stress from your body — weeds laugh when we just snip off their hair, but they cringe when we tug up their roots. Allowing "the shake," or even encouraging it to begin, goes straight to the root of tension or trauma, loosening it from the grip of the inner layers of your muscles, then elevating it up and *out* of you — body, mind, and soul.

When you experience any category of threat, your body's fight-or-flight (or freeze) response is awakened, blood is directed to your defense organs, and adrenaline floods your body, helping to protect you from the threat and keep you alive. Once the threat has passed, the body releases the built-up survival energy through shaking. I don't want you to have to wait for a mountain lion to chase you, or a stint in traffic next to a car blaring heavy metal music, for you to release pent-up survival energy. I want to empower you to claim your right to harmonized energy and a peaceful state of being *now*.

I learned the importance of surrendering to shaking when I was birthing my son. I thought I was mega-failing at birth because I could not stop my legs from shaking through the surges. For the first few hours of labor I attempted to control the shaking (because I thought it was "wrong") by applying pressure to my legs, which served only to make me feel like millions of lemmings were chipping their way out of my body with tiny ice picks. When I became too exhausted to hold back the quakes, I became high — spiritually high. Each time I shook through a surge I felt lighter and more expanded. After an hour of this I felt like I was floating above the starchy hospital sheets I was sweating through. I also noticed a freedom from the anxiety I had previously held over the final phase of birth — the pushing-a-human-out-of-a-wormhole phase.

Shaking Starter Kit

I'm not going to tell you to "just shake it off," because that saying is super annoying and diminishes your very real experience of stress. But I will tell you to welcome and accept the shaking. Shaking is sexy.

Practice the following exercises to stimulate shaking, allowing you to release pent-up stress and tension and become comfortable with surrendering to the sensations of tremors you'll likely experience during childbirth.

OPEN LOTUS

Sit up straight in bed, or on the floor with a pillow supporting your back. Bend your knees in a comfortable position with your feet resting flat on the surface in front of you.

Open lotus, initial position

Next, spread your knees about twenty inches apart, allowing the inner sides of your feet to slightly lift off the floor. Allow your knees to spread until you feel some muscular strain in your thighs. Stay in this position, without supporting your legs with anything but their own strength, until they begin to shake. Permit the tremors to continue for two to eight minutes. It is natural if the shaking elevates in intensity over time.

Open lotus, shaking position, front view

Open lotus, shaking position, side view

When you're ready for the tremors to end, lay your legs flat in front of you, allowing them to fully relax as you lightly massage them.

LYING DOWN OPEN LOTUS

Lie on your side, with one support pillow behind your back and one under your head. Bend your knees and lift them off the bed so your bottom knee is a few inches from the mattress (keep your feet resting on the bed).

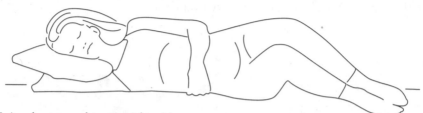

Lying down open lotus, initial position

Next, lift your top knee a few inches above your bottom knee. Stay in this position, without supporting your legs with anything but their own strength, until they begin to shake. Permit the tremors to continue for two to eight minutes.

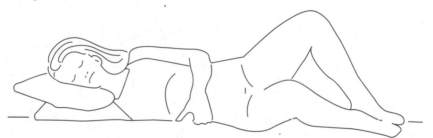

Lying down open lotus, shaking position

When you're ready for the tremors to end, lay your legs back on the bed, allowing them to fully relax as you lightly massage them.

Allow shaking for only two to eight minutes at a time to ensure you don't become overwhelmed by the sensations. Listen to your body's intuition, starting and stopping these exercises, and the resulting tremors, when you feel ready.

RIDDLE: What term means "energy force" in Chinese and is used to describe the electricity buzzing through pathways in your body?

Go to **YourSereneLife.wordpress.com/chapter-three** and use the one-word riddle answer as your offer code to download the relaxation recording for this chapter!

CALL TO PLEASURE

- Each day, practice tapping through one fear or concern: First, move through the process of meditating on what your intensity level is regarding the issue you're working on, then prepare your system by rubbing your tender spots while stating your issue, and finally, move through the ten-point tapping sequence while stating your issue-specific affirmation. Repeat the tapping sequence until your intensity level has lowered.

- Every evening, assume one of the tremor-inducing positions described above until your legs, or your entire body, begins to shake. Allow your deeply embedded tension and trauma to be released for two to eight minutes as you breathe through any resistance. (End this exercise early if you begin to feel overwhelmed.)

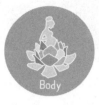

Body

CHAPTER FOUR

PRENATAL EXERCISE
From Squats to Kegels

Just Breathe: *As you take deep-in-the-belly breaths, meditate on the fact that each breath fills your muscles with energizing oxygen that will make exercise easier and more comfortable.*

Prenatal exercise upgraded me from an insecure, cranky, sex-loathing, bloated baby-making machine to a self-assured, (mostly) chipper, svelte (yet still bulging), sex-craving pregnant lady.

Before opening up my womb to guests, I exercised because I had to — it was my organic version of Valium. I forced myself to do it, trying to ignore what I was doing until I sweated enough to warrant stopping and getting in the shower. Halfway through my first trimester, something shifted and I "got it." I got how exercise spiritually connected me to my body (and now my baby). I got how pushing my body through difficult (not to be confused with painful) moves expanded my perception of my physical abilities. I got how exercise gave my mind and spirit (and Baby) jazz-hand attitudes. I also really enjoyed giving up long-distance running during pregnancy.

Speaking of long-distance running, the key to exercising regularly during pregnancy is giving up all the routines that don't make you feel good and strong in your body, in favor of practices that make you feel amazing and sexy. And yes ma'am, sex counts as exercise.

As we explore various body-movin' options in this chapter, I want you to tune in to what makes you excited. I want the flavors of exercise you resonate with to become so sacred and integral to your pregnancy that you crave them daily. When this happens, when exercise becomes your daily dose of happy, you'll be stoked to continue the ritual, even when your baby is out of the womb, strapped to your chest, and pinching your nipples.

> OBLIGATORY DISCLAIMER:
> *Talk to your medical care provider before starting any new exercise regime, stay hydrated, avoid activities that put you at risk for blunt force trauma, and rest when you feel fatigued.*

Train Your Body to Feel Good

I exercise because it gives me my daily fix of endorphins. A secondary benefit is a firm upper butt (the lower part is still saggy).

Endorphins are your body's natural pain relievers and can be up to two hundred times more powerful than morphine, when they're given the space (through deep breathing) to build upon themselves. This yummy hormone blocks your brain's ability to receive messages of pain from the sensory nerves, improves your mood, and can be passed through the placenta to Baby. The parties endorphins are most likely to attend are exercise and childbirth — two situations that require your body to temper your discomfort. But endorphins need to be trained in tempering pain. The more you exercise, the more skilled your body will become at producing and releasing endorphins. This body knowledge will filter into birth, allowing the endorphin floodgates to be opened. Heck, if your body becomes a proficient endorphin factory through prenatal exercise, the entire endorphin dam may just bust open during birth. *Now* do you feel motivated?

Change the Name, Change Your Perception

If the E-word makes you say "bleh," let's give it a different name — *nature trek, aquatic adventure, birthing prep, physical synergy, body bonding, de-gunking, happy pill replacing,* or whatever else makes you shift your attitude to more of a "yay!" than a "nay." Your mind tells your body what to do, so if your mind reacts to the word *exercise* by telling the body to reorganize the scarf collection, Google the top baby names in Sweden, and eat some chips, then we need to give it a name less likely to evoke the Art of Avoidance.

Visualize Yourself Exercising

You don't need to convince your body to exercise, just your mind. While sitting in bed every evening, close your eyes and visualize yourself joyfully moving through the exercise ritual you plan on practicing the following day. See yourself smiling through the entire practice, feeling stronger and more capable with every move, sway, or booty drop. Feel the accomplishment and vibrant energy you're coursing with as you finish. Set the intent that this is how your workout will unfold the following day, preventing your mind from sending resistance to your body when it's time to get that sexy body moving.

You Can Still CrossFit

An unofficial symptom of pregnancy is paranoia. Occasionally it's so serious a baby-loaded lady may avoid walking by the grocery store deli in fear that a whiff of the lunch meat may cause her baby to grow two heads. Exercise is another source of paranoia. (What a weird combo — exercise and lunch meat.)

Many women stop exercising altogether during the first weeks of pregnancy for fear that any bouncing or stretching will cause the uterus to dislodge the fertilized egg — unlikely. The question of prenatal exercise is one that can best be answered by your care provider. By knowing your past and current medical history, the state of your pregnancy, and the level of activity you maintained pre-pregnancy, they can assist in determining what level of activity you can safely partake in during the different stages of pregnancy. I promise they will want you to maintain some level of physical activity, with the rare exception of mamas on bed rest.

The general parameter most care providers suggest is this: if you and Baby are healthy, you can safely maintain your pre-pregnancy exercise regimen for most of your pregnancy, with the exception of activities that pose a high risk for your belly sustaining blunt force. When your belly begins to bulge, you will need to adjust any activities that require you to lie flat on your back, or that would smoosh your belly. You're no mummy-dummy; when a particular move or activity begins to feel *off*, you'll know it's time to remove it from your repertoire. With the go-ahead from your care provider, the activities described in this chapter are safe during all stages of your pregnancy.

Become the Queen of Quickies

Exercise does not have to be held together by laces, sweat-wicking spandex, and a Jillian Michaels playlist you found in a fitness magazine. Toning and stretching your muscles and livening up your heart rate can happen anyplace, anytime.

Of the suggestions below, some are a few of the endorphin-eliciting quickies I partook in while my uterus was packing a baby, and some are ideas from the human making babes I've worked with. I encourage you to try these, then work out your creative nature by thinking up new ways to get in a quickie.

- **Squats:** While you're doing dishes, scrolling through your phone, or engaging in any other stationary activity, squat into it. A squat is an excellent way to prep your birthing muscles and get comfortable assuming the most effective birthing position, which is…a squat. Play around with the squat until you find a position that you feel secure in while it's causing your glutes and thighs to tighten. No need to assume a full squat; bending your knees a bit and lowering your tush a few inches is effective. Squat for as long as you feel comfortable, and upgrade the benefits by dropping some Kegels into the mix.
- **Conquer the stairs:** There's a reason the "take the stairs" advice is repeated ad nauseam — it works. Whenever possible, forgo the awkward silence of an elevator and take the Stairway to Endorphins. And hey, Babe, be safe — hold on to the handrail, and take your time. (You can take the elevator when the baby comes out.)
- **Befriend the forgotten parking lot:** Have you ever been in an overcrowded mall parking lot during the holidays? With all those grannies and soccer moms busting out their most-lethal stares and

pushy driving maneuvers to procure The Spot? Double-dip yourself in good fortune by taking your hat out of the ring, parking in that empty lot way in the back, and getting some exercise.

- **Nest it up:** Organizing and cleaning a house in preparation for a baby isn't for sissies — it's for rad-ass women like you. If you're resisting the task of repurposing your home for a baby, try reframing the project into a form of exercise — it can motivate you to pack up your partner's rare knife collection, throw away the orphaned Tupperware lids, and learn how to use that dry mop your mother-in-law bought you last year.

- **Gab and gait:** I once got off a juicy phone call and had no idea where I was. I had walked up my street, shuffled down some side streets, and found a hiking trail — I was a mile and a half from home. Whenever you need to make a phone call, stand up and start walking — even if you're just walking in circles in your living room. Listening to your girlfriend gab about her laser hair removal debacle or your coworker bitch about Sally from the social media department will distract you from the fact that, "Hey! You're toning your butt!"

- **Stand up for your health:** Sitting is the new high-fructose corn syrup. When you sit for long periods of time, your circulation is constricted, your brain gets lethargic, and your body shifts into idle. Place your laptop on the kitchen counter, request a standing desk at work, or set a timer to go off every hour, reminding you to stand up and stretch for a few minutes. But respect the moods of your body and sit down if you begin feeling sore or fatigued — behind every healthy mama should be a comfy chair with a footstool.

- **Book walk:** I learned what to look for in a good breast pump, how to practice nonviolent communication, ways to improve my social media presence, and how to be in The Now — all while walking. There's an audiobook for everything. Utilize the power of learning (and juicy romance mystery thrillers!) to get you moving. Download a book on your phone and *only* let yourself listen to it while you're on a walk.

- **Spontaneous dance:** Life is so much better when you let yourself break out in the Carlton. If you schedule a dance break every hour,

49

where you stand up and do an inhibition-free shimmy to your favorite song, your life will never be stale.

- **Screen stretches:** Take advantage of the fact that staring at a screen can be addictive by exercising in tandem with your screen time. While you're watching that documentary on honey badgers, or the *Real Housewives* reunion, move through some gentle stretches, being sure not to overextend yourself.

Yoga

Downward Poodle, transitioned into Awkward Side-Bend, into Upward Bloated Cow, with a Queefing (a.k.a. "air blasting out of the vagina when you least expect it") Squat finale — sounds fun, right? While real yoga-ese is more eloquent, those descriptors depict how I felt at the beginning of my prenatal yoga practice — my queefing became so intense I felt like my baby was sneezing whenever I did a forward bend. Fortunately, my awkwardness during yoga eventually married a heightened state of awareness, deeper sense of connection with my baby, and a stronger core (and a *kind of* firmer butt), all of which strengthened my belief that my body could actually birth a human.

The holistic practice of Yoga originated in ancient India as long ago as 3000 BCE. Varieties of Yoga are studied in Buddhism, Hinduism, and Jainism, and it has been steadily growing in popularity in the West for the past several decades. This is one trend that has refused to go out of style, and for good reason.

Below are a few pregnancy-safe moves to get you started. To dig further, find a local prenatal yoga class or buy a prenatal yoga DVD. Before beginning, read through the following safety considerations:

- If you would like to move through all of the poses in "one go," slowly move into one pose, hold for thirty to sixty seconds, then return to a relaxed standing position (or cross-legged sitting position for floor poses) before moving into the next pose.
- Transition out of a pose before thirty to sixty seconds are up if you feel unreasonable discomfort or instability (or you "gotta go").

- Practice all standing poses next to a secure chair that you can utilize for stability, if needed.
- Be sure to perform all poses on a well-padded yoga mat for proper support.

Energizing Side-Angle Pose

Opens your hips, stretches your side, and releases your reserves of fresh chi (life force).

Energizing side-angle pose

    Ease into a comfortable right-legged lunge and rest your right elbow on your right thigh. Keeping your torso open to the left, extend your left arm over your head and gaze at the fingertips of your left hand. Hold for thirty to sixty seconds, return to a standing position, and repeat on the left side.

Balancing Triangle Pose

Strengthens your legs, stretches your side, enhances your balance, and opens your heart center.

    Stand with your feet four to five feet apart, keeping your heels aligned. Turn your right foot out to the right in a ninety-degree angle, and slightly pivot your left foot toward your right. Raise your arms out to your side until they're parallel to the floor. Keeping your arms straight, reach your right

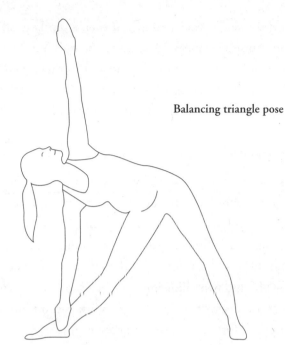

Balancing triangle pose

hand down to rest on your right shin, right ankle, or the floor by your right foot. Gaze up at your left hand, which is reaching toward the sky. Hold for thirty to sixty seconds, slowly return to a standing position, and repeat on the left side.

Spacious Side Stretch

Expands your waist, pelvis, and hips and provides more room for Baby by helping to elongate your torso.

Stand with your feet side by side on the floor. Reach your arms above your head, keeping them straight but not locking your elbows, and interlace your fingers, allowing your index

Spacious side stretch

fingers to point toward the sky. Inhale, and as you exhale gently push your left hip to the side and your upper torso and arms to the right until you feel a light stretch in your left side. Focus on lifting up and through your arms and spine, and avoid jutting your hip too far out to the left. Hold for thirty to sixty seconds, then return to center and repeat on other side.

Spine-Strengthening Cat-Cow Pose

Relieves and prevents back pain and eases Baby away from your spine.

Begin with your hands and knees on the floor, ensuring your knees are directly under your hips; and your wrists, directly under your shoulders. With your spine neutral, inhale, and as you exhale round your back up, relaxing your neck and tucking your chin toward your chest. As you inhale again, slowly arch your back down, allowing your belly to relax as you lift your chin and tailbone up toward the sky. Allow your breath to guide you through at least ten cycles before ending with a neutral spine.

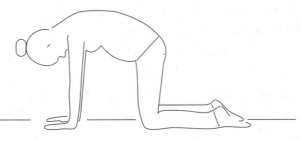

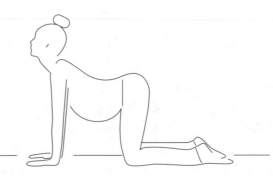

Spine-strengthening cat-cow pose

Kneading Kneel

Massages and stretches the arches in your feet, and increases circulation to your frequently used, yet forgotten, tootsies.

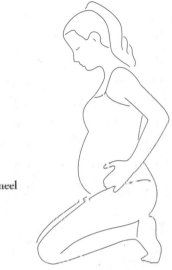

Kneading kneel

Kneel on the floor with your heels resting in the flesh of your booty and your toes tucked under, pointed toward your knees. Place a pillow under your knees, if needed.

Lengthening Toe Stretch

Works to stretch and strengthen your core, butt, back, arms, and legs.

Sit on the floor with your right leg stretched out straight and your left leg bent, with the left heel resting against your right thigh. Grip the toes of

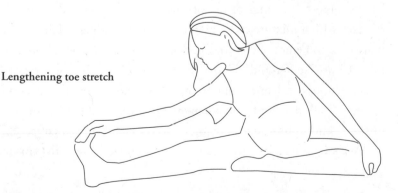

Lengthening toe stretch

your right foot with your right hand, then gently pull your toes toward you while focusing on extending your right leg and heel away from you. Keep your chest open to your left. Hold for thirty to sixty seconds, return to an erect seated position, and repeat on the other side.

Gas-Relieving Child's Pose

Helps you relax enough to fart!

Kneel down in front of a large pillow (e.g., a couch pillow) or a stack of bedroom pillows. Place one or two additional pillows under your hips for support, then lean forward until your head is resting on the pillow. Wrap your arms around the pillow in the position that is most comfortable. Add more pillows, or reposition your body, if you feel any uncomfortable strain in your body. Rest here until you're ready to resume activity.

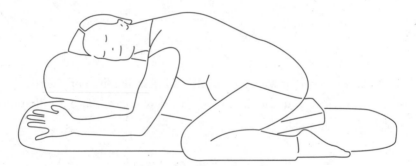

Gas-relieving child's pose

Walking

I awoke most mornings of my pregnancy feeling like I'd been splashed in the face with a mixture of all six pregnancy hormones. I felt nervous, tired, nauseous, and emotionally whacked. On these mornings, before I could talk myself into Netflix and all-you-can-eat cereal, I forced my robot body to change out of the flannels, put on my tennis shoes, slip my book on CD into my sexy Walkman, and grab a banana on my way out the door. Within ten minutes, endorphins made me forget how much I missed coffee.

Walking is free, it's easy, and it gets you outside. Fresh air is kryptonite to negative energy, empowering all your yummy feel-good hormones to come out and play. Walking also supplies extra oxygen to you and Baby and removes you from a potentially stale indoor atmosphere. And it encourages you to whoosh.

What's that? You haven't whooshed? Do it now: inhale, then exhale the word *whoosh*, and feel a release. Hear that sound in your mind's ear as you walk, visualizing negativity whooshing out of you with each step. The whoosh can also be an effective tool for encouraging Baby to turn into the vertex (head-down) position — as you walk, envision Baby's head whooshing down to nestle into your lower pelvic region. Walk on a stable and flat path, wear supportive shoes, and bring a fully charged cell phone in case you need backup.

Swimming

Immersing your pregnant Self in warm water offers you a glimpse into the weightless world Baby is playing in. Feeling your body slide through the smooth anatomy of water connects you to both your baby and your innate fluidity.

Propelling yourself through water is also the ultimate prebirth meditation. Before you step into the water, ask it to heal, cleanse, and support you, and as you enter give the water a few moments to adjust its frequency to the channel of love. As you move through the water, set up your birthing muscles for ultimate pliability during birth by envisioning the essence of water seeping into your mind, body, and spirit. Set the intention that your whole being will become more adept at displaying its fluid nature each time you go for a swim. Settle into a stroke so rhythmic you no longer have to consciously think about your movements — you can just *be*. Each time you swim you'll be setting yourself up for a smooth and comfortable birth experience.

Engage in this all-inclusive form of exercise by traveling to a local (and safe!) body of water, or joining your local athletic club. Aquatic meditation whilst listening to water-aerobic jams at a YMCA will prepare you for trying to meditate with kids around.

Here is a full-body water routine that will take thirty to forty-five minutes:

- Five laps of walking or running in the shallow end.
- Fifty reps of scissors kicks: Standing up straight, lift your right leg up in front of you until it creates a ninety-degree angle with your left leg. Hold for a moment, lower your right leg, and repeat the sequence with your left leg. Switch back and forth for fifty reps.
- Twenty-five jumping jacks in water that is up to your waist.
- Ten to fifteen slow and steady laps in the pool, using whatever stroke you feel most comfortable with.
- Rest by floating in the water with your eyes closed for twenty deep breaths.

Vaginal Strengthening

Blessings of a Perky Vagina: Better orgasms, more efficient laboring muscles, speedier postpartum recovery, urinary control, and did I mention better orgasms?

Pelvic floor exercises, called Kegels, are unexpectedly satisfying and can be done anywhere — the car, the shower, in bed, while mopping, while nursing, while gossiping, during sex, at work, right here, and over there.

Your pelvic floor knows what's up, and how to keep it there. It supports your uterus, bladder, small intestines, and rectum. Have you ever heard the common postpartum sentiment, "I felt like my insides were going to fall out after giving birth"? That's not an encouraging statement for a pregnant woman! While your innards are unlikely to slip out, you may experience a postpartum drooping sensation in your nether regions, which Kegels will help combat.

How to Squeeze Out Those Reps

1. Identify your pelvic floor muscles by stopping your stream of urine midflow (release after a few seconds).
2. Focus on pulling the pelvic floor muscles in and up, hold for the count of ten, and then fully release to the count of ten.
3. During release, be cognizant of the sensation of relaxing these muscles and take a mental note of *how* you're releasing them. The full release is the sensation you'll want to focus on during birth.

4. During reps, maintain smooth and easy breathing: slowly inhaling with the intake of muscles, and exhaling with the release.
5. Meditate on the results you seek to gain during each Kegel — effective birth surges, comfortable labor, intact perineum, and so on.

Do ten sets, three times a day.

Kegels are funny — go ahead and giggle when you're Kegel-ing in unorthodox vagina-strengthening locations.

From Her Heart to Yours

Exercise kept me from having an emotional breakdown. I never experienced morning sickness, just morning meltdowns. I would wake up each day feeling like the weight of humanity was pressing on my chest, and I would cry — not cute tears but loud, wracking sobs. I called my care provider on one of these mornings, after cracking open an egg with a double yoke. (I was eating twins!) My midwife was busy, but her receptionist recommended I take a walk around the block. I walked around my block, then another and another until I stopped crying and felt energized. Exercise had never been "my thing" before, but it was the only act that could quell my unexplained sadness. I began walking two miles every morning, sometimes crying, sometimes not. After a few weeks, the aching emotion in my chest was replaced by a light and expanded sensation. Now, when my baby cries, I strap her to my chest and we walk.

— *S. J., Santa Cruz, California*

RIDDLE: What type of exercise helps you feel what Baby may be feeling in utero?

Go to **YourSereneLife.wordpress.com/chapter-four** and use the one-word riddle answer as your offer code to download the relaxation recording for this chapter!

CALL TO PLEASURE

- Check with your care provider to determine any exercise limitations you need to honor.
- Each day, incorporate three of the "quickie" exercises listed.
- For one week, rotate between yoga, walking, swimming, and any other type of exercise you feel drawn to. Meditate on which one (or maybe more than one) you sync with, and set a commitment to practice your chosen exercise(s) for a total of forty-five minutes a day, five days a week.
- Mentally recite five things you love about your body each day.
- Do ten sets of Kegels, three times a day.

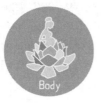

CHAPTER FIVE

THE NOURISHING BASICS
What to Eat

Just Breathe: Infuse your belly with ten deep breaths, envisioning your digestive system becoming more receptive to nutrients with each inhalation, and releasing toxins with every exhalation.

Contrary to the seductive "pregnant-gluttony" the media often touts, you're not eating for yourself and a linebacker. You're eating for yourself and a growing ball of cells, and those cells only need around three hundred additional calories each day. While the amount of food you eat during pregnancy will not dramatically change, the *way* you eat will shift. My goal for you is not that you become proficient at counting calories and sticking to a strict pregnancy diet. The intention of this chapter is to awaken your innate ability to forge a harmonious relationship with food and appreciate the gifts it offers.

Oneness is the root of harmony. When you feel unity with the food you eat you'll organically settle into balanced eating habits. Before putting food in your mouth, ask yourself, "Do I feel unity with this food? Will it nourish me?" If you falter in answering and don't feel great about putting it in your mouth, don't do it. Sometimes, you'll feel *really good* about putting that piece of chocolate cheesecake in your mouth, and that's great! You can absolutely savor the occasional treat.

Guilt is often floating around the periphery of our meals. To dissolve negative connotations (and habits) commonly attached to food, reframe your perception of food from "guilty pleasure" to "baby-building blocks." When you imagine each bite you take becoming a Lego-like addition to your developing baby, food takes on a sacred nature, moving you to a space where you naturally (and happily) select the healthiest fare (most of the time).

Poetic Eating

When you shift your perception of food from something that needs to be shoved in your mouth so you can move on to the next activity, to morsels of poetry you have the pleasure of slowly noticing and relishing, your loving relationship with food is born. Allow words of detailed appreciation to scroll through your mind as each bite enters your mouth.

For example, "This avocado feels smooth and rich in my mouth. The seasoning coating it enhances the creamy flavors and creates enhanced salivation. As the avocado slides down my throat, I feel my body absorbing its nutrients and passing them to my baby. Thank you, avocado — you're mega-yummy."

This practice also encourages you to eat more slowly, providing your body time to send signals to your mind that it is satiated, before you overeat and awaken latent heartburn. Fight heartburn with poetry.

Eat for Your Body, Not Your Mind

The hungry pregnant mind can be chaotic, barking out orders to eat the entire bag of potato chips — "Because I'm tired, and potato chips will make me feel better." When this occurs, it's often because the mind has disconnected from the needs of the body. When you feel the mental barking commence, allow your body to take the reins from your mind before you begin eating.

You can do this via a body scan that takes about thirty seconds:

1. Close your eyes and focus on your breath.
2. Notice (without judgment) the thoughts in your mind, then allow your attention to float down and away from the head.
3. Scan down until you land on the part of the body that is expressing

hunger (likely your stomach, or maybe your elbow?), then ask what it's hungry for. If possible, feed it what it wants.

During this scan you may notice that there is *not* an area of your body expressing hunger; it's only your mind. If this is the case, ask the mind what it needs (with the exception of food) to settle. Maybe you need to cry, or walk around, or rest, or drink some water. When food is consumed for the mind and not the body, overeating of unnourishing food often occurs. The most common catalyst for this mind-eating is fatigue — our mind easily confuses the need for a nap with a need for a cheeseburger.

Daily Essentials

With rare exceptions, healthy, well-nourished mothers birth healthy babies. In addition to minimizing the occurrence of toxemia, pre-eclampsia, mal-positioned babies, and the need for interventions during birthing, balanced nutrition creates a strong mama, who sprouts a healthy baby, who is better equipped to play his role in easier birthing. Wholesome eating also shifts the chemistry of your body, releases the optimal prescription of hormones, spices up your libido, and carves vitality into the rest of your baby's life.

Here are general guidelines to follow as you craft your daily meals (after passing any shifts in your dietary plan by your care provider). To reduce the level of chemicals your baby is exposed to, buy the organic version of all foods listed below, when possible.

Protein

Everyone and their health-magazine-reading cousin will tell you protein is the boss lady when it comes to pregnancy nutrition. Protein sticks its nose in every critical function of the body and needs to be replenished on the regular. If you consume 75 to 115 grams of protein a day, taken in several snacks or light meals (protein should account for one-quarter to one-third of your daily food intake), you'll maintain healthy weight gain, lower your chances of developing gestational diabetes, support the health of your uterus and placenta, lower the chances of birth defects, enhance the cognitive activity and growth in your baby's brain, and start to sprout wings (in your mind).

- **Great sources of protein:** Eggs! Daily! Cottage cheese, lean meats, fish (salmon is a "Yay!"), cheese (with the exception of unpasteurized cheese; ask your care provider for a list of all the delicious foods they don't want you to eat), tofu, nuts, beans (always have lentil soup in the fridge!), milk, yogurt, and cream cheese.
- **Surprising sources of protein:** Sundried tomatoes, guava, artichokes, and peas.

Green

Green food is the resident goddess of pregnant nutrition. The essential nutrients found in many green vegetables (e.g., vitamins A, C, E, and K, antioxidants, calcium, iron, folate, riboflavin, folic acid!, magnesium, and beta-carotene) support the immune system, healthy vision, cell and tissue development, and healthy bones and teeth. They also offer virus and infection protection, controlled blood pressure, a reduction of your risk of anemia, and many more delicious benefits. And shamrock marshmallows dipped in green food dye don't count.

- **Great sources of green:** Avocados are so fine, eat them often and your body and baby will thank you. Their healthy fats help build your baby's skin, brain, and tissues. Under the avocado, load your plate with green leafy vegetables, green beans, broccoli, asparagus, peas, squash, peppers, celery, cabbage, bok choy, kale, chard, and other green things that come from the earth. Because chewing on foliage can become tiresome, throw a few of these options in a smoothie, and ask your care provider about safe green-powder mixes (containing goodies like spirulina, acai, aloe, and more) you can add to drinks.

Orange and Yellow

Orange and yellow fare is the strength-and-endurance trainer of pregnancy sustenance. Foods with a sunny flare are chockablock full of antioxidants, fiber, vitamins, and phytonutrients that nourish your heart, eyes, and skin while protecting you and Baby from harmful bacteria, viruses, and other yuck. These foods provide three essential nutrients: beta-carotene (can delay cognitive aging and protect skin from sun damage), vitamin A (supports Baby's embryonic growth, helps with postpartum tissue repair, boosts the immune system, and can neutralize damaging free radicals), and vitamin C (reduces risk of cardiovascular disease, rebuilds tissue, heals wounds, supports bone growth, and boosts the immune system). Some additional goodies are flavonoids, lycopene, potassium, and zeaxanthin! Phew!

- **Great sources of orange and yellow:** Carrots, butternut and spaghetti squashes, bell peppers, papayas, cantaloupes, pumpkins, yellow beets, corn (roasted with some ghee, lemon pepper, and sea salt!), bananas, mangoes, yams, sweet potatoes (can help remineralize teeth), oranges (help to prevent neural tube defects), peaches, apricots, persimmons, grapefruit, and lemons (help to balance pH levels and yummy on apples).

Fruits and Berries

These are the iron (wo)men of pregnancy nutrients. Many fruits and berries are high in vitamin C, which helps the body absorb iron. (Good iron levels keep your energy levels up!) These colorful little treats are also packed with water, good carbs, antioxidants, fiber, and plant compounds.

- **Great sources of fruity-berry goodness:** Strawberries, blueberries (extra credit for these), honeydew melons, watermelons, raspberries, kiwis, grapes, apples, pineapples, pears, and any other fresh fruit finds you can score at your local farmers' market. Fresh fruit is the best (or frozen fruit for smoothies), but if you would like to snack on dried fruit, ensure it was not made with added sugar.

Fiber

Fiber is the cleanup crew of pregnancy cuisine — it keeps everything moving, sweeping unneeded gunk down and out of the body and helping to prevent the delights of heartburn, constipation, indigestion, and overeating along the way. It also helps ward off hemorrhoids! Fiber's résumé also includes prevention of glucose intolerance (which can segue into gestational diabetes), reduction of your risk for pre-eclampsia, and diminution of your chance of developing cervical or ovarian cancer.

- **Great sources of fiber:** Most fruits, vegetables, and whole grains will provide fiber, but here are a few of my favorites that offer a mega-dose of the rough stuff: lentils, peas, beans, chickpeas (canned chickpeas tossed in coconut oil, salt, and pepper, then baked, are yum yum), soybeans, peanuts, chia and flax seeds (great smoothie additions), artichokes, broccoli, Brussels sprouts, avocados, pears, raspberries, and apples.

Whole Grains

Intact grains are the foundation of pregnancy nutrients. They are humming with nutrients: iron (prevents the condition of having too few red blood cells that can make you feel tired and cause Baby to be born too small or too early), selenium (helps to regulate immune and thyroid function), and magnesium (supports the prevention of poor fetal growth, pre-eclampsia, and infant mortality). Whole grains also offer a wallop of nutrients (e.g., vitamins B_1 and B_2, folic acid, and niacin) your babe needs to build pretty much every part of her body, and the placenta, your new organ that supports her life.

- **Great sources of whole grains:** Steel-cut oats (load them with fruit and fiber-full seeds!), barley, quinoa (a god in the whole grain world!), French or sourdough bread, corn on the cob, brown rice, whole-wheat pita pockets, buckwheat, spelt, and air-popped popcorn. Look for products that are "100% whole grain" (nothing "refined" or "enriched").

Water

Water is the breath of pregnancy nutrition — without it, nothing else can move around, be absorbed, or survive. Water prevents dehydration, which can lead to nausea, headaches, cramps, edema, and dizziness, and it is so important I have honored it with its own chapter, beginning on page 122. Amp up your water intake during your third trimester, when dehydration can cause contractions and spark preterm labor. Starting *now*, drink around one hundred ounces of water each day — twelve to thirteen 8-ounce cups of water.

- **Great sources of water:** The tap in your kitchen (make sure it's thoroughly filtered), coconut water, skim milk, sparkling water, fruit and vegetables juices without added sugar, and decaffeinated tea.

Omega-3 Fish Oil

Omega-3 fatty acids are the go-to smarties of pregnancy nutrients. A family of long-chain polyunsaturated fatty acids, they are crucial for Baby's health and development, as well as your own. The leaders of omega-3s are EPA (nourisher of the heart, immune system, and inflammatory response) and DHA (supporter of the brain, eyes, and central nervous system). Most types of fish provide a helping of omega-3s, but beware of fish that contains high mercury levels, like tuna, shark, and swordfish. Avoid all raw fish and oysters. We dive deeper into omega-3 on the next page.

- **Great sources of omega-3 fish oil:** Salmon (improves antioxidant defenses), sardines (not as bad as you think), and purified fish oil supplements (ask your care provider what brands they recommend).

Salt

Salt is not the enemy when you use a happy option like Himalayan pink salt, which creates an electrolyte balance, increases hydration, regulates water content inside and outside cells, balances pH, reduces acid reflux, prevents muscle cramping, strengthens bones, lowers blood pressure, and supports the metabolism. *And* it's pink.

Calcium

Calcium is like the framework (or skeleton!) of pregnancy nutrition — it supports the healthy construction and growth of Baby's teeth, bones, heart, nerves, and muscles, in addition to boosting Baby's blot-clotting abilities and healthy heart rhythm. Calcium is a critical nutrient to get enough of: if you're in short supply, your body will pull calcium from your bones and teeth, then pass it on to Baby, eventually leaving you with a lower bone mass if you don't reload. Eat your collard greens! Or avocados. Or Brazil nuts. Or...

> FUN FACT! *Fermented and naturally sour food (like citrus fruit) and beverages take away sugar cravings.*

- **Great sources of calcium:** Low-fat dairy, beans, figs, okra, turnip greens, almonds, collard greens, avocados, and Brazil nuts.

Daily Servings Guide

- **Protein:** Two to three servings (1 serving = 3 ounces, or the size of a deck of cards)
- **Green:** Two servings (1 serving = 1 cup)
- **Orange and yellow:** Three servings (1 serving = ½ cup)
- **Fruits and berries:** Two to three servings (1 serving = ½ cup)
- **Fiber-rich foods (legumes, nuts, etc.):** Two to three servings (1 serving = ½ cup) for 25 to 35 grams of fiber per day
- **Whole grains:** Three servings (1 serving = ½ cup or 1 slice)
- **Water:** About 100 ounces of water each day, or twelve to thirteen 8-ounce cups of water
- **Omega-3 fish oil:** Daily, take a high-quality fish oil supplement that has at least 300 mg of DHA. Or every week have at least two servings of an omega-3-rich fish that has low levels of mercury (1 serving = 3 ounces, or the size of a deck of cards).
- **Salt:** To taste
- **Calcium:** 1,000 mg per day

Don't stuff yourself to meet these requirements, but *do* select dietary options that fulfill one or more of these essentials over foods with empty calories (e.g., processed foods with white sugar or flour).

MEGA-MAMA SMOOTHIE RECIPE

To start your day with an epic dose of wellness, blend up these here beauties:

8 ounces almond milk
Splash of coconut water
½ banana
1 teaspoon bee pollen
2 teaspoons ground flaxseed
2 teaspoons chia seeds
2 tablespoons hemp seeds
1 tablespoon cacao nibs

1 tablespoon green powder (check with your care provider on what
   they recommend)

1 pitted date (Note: According to a study published in the *Journal
   of Obstetrics and Gynecology*, women who ate a date a day for
   the entirety of their pregnancy were more dilated when their
   labor began, had less need for artificial induction, and on
   average had fewer hours of labor than women who did not eat
   dates.)

½ cup frozen blueberries

½ cup spinach

A few cubes of frozen mango

I recommend premixing a week's worth of the dry ingredients and stor-
ing the mixture in the freezer. Then, each morning mix ½ cup of the mixture
with the fruits, spinach, and liquids.

Food Fuels Endorphins!

Endorphins are not simply birthed when they sense discomfort (e.g., exercise
and childbirth); they require special ingredients to be birthed — just like
your baby. Endorphins are birthed from fats and sugar in the pituitary gland
and hypothalamus. Because endorphins require fat and sugar, you must keep
your body fueled if you want to feel good. There is a reason why a drop in
blood sugar is accompanied by lethargy and discontent. Keep the labor and
delivery unit in your body pumping out endorphin babies by supplying your
body with small and regular protein-rich meals that are short on refined
sugars and carbohydrates.

Eater Beware

Because you're one wise woman, I don't need to wax on about restrictions.
Here's a brief "Just Say No!" list for ya:

- Alcohol, cigarettes, and caffeine
- Fast food, fried food, and carnival food (I'm looking at you, funnel
   cakes.)

- The Whites: Limit refined sugar, white-flour products, white rice, and white potatoes.

Of course, you deserve the occasional treat — as long as your indulgence doesn't include a shot of tequila with a side of cigarette, you can periodically satisfy your need for sweet. When you do, slow down, savor each bite, and soak in the experience so you don't need to go back for more, and more, and then the whole box.

Oh, and avoiding the bad and feasting on the good will help prevent the "S-word": stretch marks.

From Her Heart to Yours

Pregnancy turned me into a competitive eater with a proclivity for barfing because I was being told, "You're eating for two! Have some more! Indulge yourself!" I would stuff my face with *all the things* — until I threw up. I ate so quickly my body didn't have time to alert my mind to incoming disaster before I had eaten one too many slices of cheese and was lifting up the toilet seat. I feared my meals.

Then in my childbirth preparation class we discussed the rule of "six small and intentional rainbow meals a day." We were encouraged to meditate for three minutes before each meal, creating the space for our body to tell us what it was craving, then *slowly* prepare and eat the food (ensuring it represented a few rich colors of the rainbow), pausing after each bite to give the body time to process, then send the signal of satiation to the mind. I began enjoying and appreciating food, instead of seeing it as a vehicle for indulgence. I even developed a love for cooking — much to the joy of my partner.

— *Y. O., Los Angeles, California (mama to "three under three"!)*

RIDDLE: What is found in foods like flaxseed and lentils and "sweeps out" gunk from your body?

Go to **YourSereneLife.wordpress.com/chapter-five** and use the one-word riddle answer as your offer code to download the relaxation recording for this chapter!

CALL TO PLEASURE

- Follow these steps before each meal:

    1. Close your eyes and focus on your breath.
    2. Notice (without judgment) the thoughts in your mind, then allow your attention to float down and away from the mind.
    3. Scan down until you land on the part of the body that is expressing hunger, then ask it what it's hungry for. If possible, feed it what it wants, not what the mind is asking for.

- Make poetry out of food. In your mind, describe the flavors, textures, and aromas of each bite.
- Eat six small and intentional (and bright!) meals each day, utilizing protein-rich foods, greens, orange and yellow fruits and veggies, fresh fruits and berries, fiber-full foods, whole grains, and calcium as the building blocks for your meals.
- Drink at least 100 ounces of water each day — twelve to thirteen 8-ounce cups of water.

CHAPTER SIX

DISSOLVING FEAR THROUGH ACCEPTANCE

JUST BREATHE: *Fear is dissolved by deep breath. Take in a deep and powerful breath to a slow count of ten, envisioning your fears being gathered together in a ball as you breathe in. Then envision this ball of fear being carried out of your body as you exhale to the slow count of ten.*

A reverence is owed to fear — it holds the power to veer us away from danger and it provides us opportunities to discover and claim our courage, allowing us to grow in ways impossible to access without a powerful impetus. So thanks, fear — we honor you. Now we're going to learn how to get you the heck out of our way.

Fear can be a catalyst for growth only when it is acknowledged and accepted, then shown the door. When it becomes a festering guest it begins swallowing up your reserves of health, happiness, and sanity, sticking you in a "what-if" paralysis. The oftentimes-*false* illusions that give birth to fear (e.g., a misconception that your body doesn't know how to build and birth a baby) are frequently left unchecked in the vulnerable heart, mind, and body of the pregnant mama. You may believe the fears are there to protect you, maybe to "prepare you for the worst." But instead of helping you prepare for an unlikely and unwanted outcome, the stress produced by these fears often *creates* the unwanted outcomes, like pregnancy complications, medical interventions, or postpartum depression.

The unknown sound you hear at night is much scarier than opening the door, peering outside, and seeing that the sound is just your cat chasing its tail. You're going to open the door and get to know fear. You're going to observe it, chat with it, and befriend it so it's no longer the hidden demon you run from, but a known entity you know how to communicate with, know how to kindly ask to leave when it has served its purpose. The first step is exploring the basic (illusory) anatomy of fear, and how it affects your very real physical anatomy.

The Mind-Body Effects of Fear

The skeleton of fear is composed of thoughts about a perceived (not usually real) threat. The flesh of fear is composed of the unpleasant emotions triggered by those thoughts.

As soon as a fear is birthed in your mind, the amygdala (a nut-shaped organ in the core of your brain) sends a wake-up signal to your autonomic nervous system, causing your body to acknowledge the fear. The two lanes of the autonomic nervous system, the sympathetic and parasympathetic nervous systems, are the boss ladies regulating your internal organs, telling them what to do in times of danger and peace. But sometimes, they get a little confused.

Without the sympathetic nervous system (the Panic Room), you might pet a great white shark. Without the parasympathetic nervous system (the Meditation Room), you might have a panic attack when the waiter brings you a salad instead of a hamburger. The confounding thing is, the chemical response created in the body when facing either the shark or the salad is the same, even though one has the potential to cause death, while the other is just inconvenient. Death and inconvenience both sound unpleasant, but they're way different. Unfortunately, the body does not know that they're not rated the same on the scale of seriousness.

Sympathetic Nervous System: The Panic Room

When you're shoved into the Panic Room, you fight, take flight, or freeze. Because it is unlikely you will be in many situations where physically fighting is an appropriate (or legal) response, the modern-day "fight" mechanism is to experience anxiety. A few other fun features of your Panic Room are a triggering of stress, an increase in blood pressure and heart rate, a slowing of digestion, a rerouting of blood to defense organs (the uterus is not a defense organ), and a decrease in your ability to think and reason. Fun, right? But remember, your body is not very good at deciphering an actual threat (a rattlesnake staring at you) from a perceived threat (the grocery store not having the right brand of almond milk); both situations can throw you into your Panic Room.

When you're moving through childbirth, a process that is natural and rarely life threatening, the mind often sends the body into the Panic Room because it doesn't know what to do with birth. "This is an unknown, this is scary — I don't know what to do with this. Yup, we're probably going to die." None of these thoughts are based in reality, yet they evoke a very real response in the body, making birth more challenging, and ironically, more dangerous. The quickest way to achieve a room reassignment, from the Panic Room to Meditation Room, is deep breathing, which we'll explore further in chapter 17.

Parasympathetic Nervous System: The Meditation Room

You should be living in your Meditation Room for about 98 percent of your life. You *deserve* to be living in your Meditation Room for 98 percent of your life. This is your restful space, where you get to feel all warm, fuzzy, and Zen-like. When you're living in this space you calmly respond to non–life threatening stressors, your body is at ease, all your organs (including the uterus!) are receiving the ideal amount of blood and oxygen, your breathing is slow and steady, and you feel really good. With the release and absence of fear comes entry into your Meditation Room. Delivering your baby in this Meditation Room encourages gentle, comfortable, and healthy (maybe even blissful!) birthing.

An important component of preventing your fears from pulling you out of your Meditation Room is letting them speak their piece so they can leave you be.

Give a Voice to Your Fears

Tense situations are commonly diffused after both parties freely express their opinions. Conflicts with fears are no different — your fears need a nonjudgmental space in which to express themselves before they feel compelled to move on. That space is created when you stop trying to "fix" or overcome a fear, and just sit with it in a private location. Breathe into the emotions and sensations that emerge as you allow the fear to be there. Notice them and name them. For example, "I'm breathing into the tightness I feel in my chest when I think about my fear of pushing my baby out. I'm not trying to make it go away — it's there — I'm just acknowledging it."

Resist the temptation to validate, discredit, or conquer the fear — just be present with it. As if you're watching a movie, observe the thoughts and images that come up as the fear moves through you; none of it is wrong. Any resistance, tightness, sadness, shaking, shame, pressure, anger, or any other form of emotional or physical expression is perfect, because that's what's coming up. It all has to come up to be released, and this can all happen in ninety seconds.

Ninety-Second Release

It takes ninety seconds or less for an emotion to be generated, chemically flow through the body, and be set free. If you say, "No! I do not want to feel sad right now. I'm going to force myself to feel something else," and resist the ninety-second surge of sadness, you'll need to process it again and again until you surrender to it. You can handle anything for ninety seconds; set your timer and breathe through it. Did you know surges during active labor often last about ninety seconds, commonly peaking at around thirty seconds, then diminishing?

How to Liberate Your Fears

Suppressing fear-induced emotions infuses life into them, often causing a manifestation of depression or unpleasant physical symptoms. Here is a plan to liberate the emotions surrounding your fears so they can have their moment and then go bother someone else:

1. Meditate on the various elements of your life (e.g., friends, family, career, body, home, incoming childbirth, etc.) and any fears that may have latched onto them.

2. Write down the fears. If you've made it this far, tremendous progress has already been made. Fears hold the greatest power when they exist without you knowing it.

3. Choose the fear that's causing you the greatest struggle and move through the following steps. There's no need to move through your entire list of fears in one day, so be gentle with yourself, creating time for rest in between fear-release sessions.

4. Set a timer for ninety seconds, close your eyes, visualize the fear, and allow the emotions attached to it to be expressed. Let yourself notice and experience the emotions and accompanying physical sensations moving through you — let go of resistance and judgment toward the fear. Hold the intention that the emotions attached to the fear will be flushed out of you by the time your alarm chimes.

   The fear you're working with may be triggered at another time. That is normal — just give yourself the ninety seconds to re-release the attached emotions.

5. Now that you've released the emotions attached to the fear, examine the fear objectively and decide where it sits on the following spectrum:

   - The object of the fear is something completely outside your control, and so the fear can be fully released by doing the ninety-second release work anytime it comes up. (This is because there is no benefit in stewing over a potential outcome you have no control over.)

   - The thing you fear is an issue you need to educate yourself on. (Knowledge gained pushes away uncertainty, and invites in confidence.) For example, I was fearful of testing positive for Group B strep, an infection caused by a common bacterium and often found in pregnancy. I educated myself on what Group B strep actually is (not as scary as I thought), and what my options would be if I tested positive. When I did test positive, I felt calm and prepared.

- The fear is something you need to talk through with another individual. Honest communication fosters peace, harmony, and connection. For example, if you're fearful of how your romantic relationship will shift after birth, share these concerns with your partner.

6. Do the work, Mama. Just do it. When you release the emotions that hold up your fears and release the fear that they will poke their heads up again (which they may do), you live from a space of love and trust, rather than one of suffering and doubt.

Do It Daily

Every morning before you get out of bed, clear any negativity that may have made itself known as you slept: close your eyes and envision any and all fears, doubts, or stressors being pulled from your mind, body, and spirit and collecting in a bubble floating in front of you. Then deeply inhale, and as you exhale imagine the bubble being blown away from you and picked up by the wind. Imagine it being pulled so far out on the horizon that it becomes a miniscule dot that pops, dissolving everything the bubble carried. Now smile, open your eyes, and claim your fresh day.

You Are Brave Enough

Intentionally inviting your fears out to play can be painful, scary, and rich with tears, but the freedom you gain when your fears have been unchained from you is immeasurable. *You are courageous enough* to awaken the inner vibrant, sumptuous, and goddess Self you probably didn't even know was waiting to spring forth. Be her, by realizing you already are her — all you need to do is take off the veil of fear.

From My Heart to Yours

When I became pregnant, life suddenly became so precious to me — specifically the life of my child. I cherished his fragile life so deeply I strangled the idea of it with fear that I would do something to screw it up. There were no empty spaces in my experience, no spaces to be filled with fun and joy and exploration — just fear. At first, I perceived this fear as love, and I was so proud to love my child so deeply. But then, when I realized enjoyment was a scant ingredient in my pregnancy, I knew I had to re-examine my definition of love.

To remove the blade of fear I had deeply embedded in my pregnancy, I forced myself to feel the blade. I had just learned of the ninety-second emotion-release work and spent an afternoon huddled in my bed with a box of tissues, allowing myself to imagine and *feel* the worst-case scenarios involving my baby, which I had been killing myself to avoid. Oh man, it hurt so bad! I brought each one up, one at a time, and gave my heart the space to ache, my eyes the space to flood, and my body the space to shake. Then, I fell asleep. I slept for thirteen hours and woke up free. My life was no longer lodged in a dark fantasy of what might happen. I was now living what was happening *in that moment*: my baby and I sitting together as one, looking out the window, noticing the Great Love that had settled in the vacant space left by fear.

— *Bailey Gaddis, Ojai, California (your authoress)*

RIDDLE: How many seconds does it take for an emotion to be generated, chemically flow through the body, and be set free?

Go to **YourSereneLife.wordpress.com/chapter-six** and use the numerical riddle answer as your offer code to download the relaxation recording for this chapter!

CALL TO PLEASURE (FEAR RELEASE)

1. Meditate on the various elements of your life (e.g., friends, family, career, body, home, incoming childbirth, etc.) and any fears that may be latched onto them.

2. Write down the fears.

3. Choose the fear that's causing you the greatest struggle.

4. Set a timer for ninety seconds, close your eyes, visualize the fear you have identified, and allow the emotions attached to it to be expressed. Let yourself notice and experience the emotions and accompanying physical sensations moving through you. Let go of resistance and judgment toward the fear. Hold the intention that the emotions attached to the fear will be flushed out of you by the time your alarm chimes.

5. Now that you've released the emotions attached to the fear, examine the fear objectively and where it sits on the following spectrum:

   • The object of the fear is something completely outside your control, so you can fully release the fear by doing the ninety-second release work anytime it comes up.

   • The thing you fear is an issue you need to educate yourself on. (Knowledge gained pushes away uncertainty and invites in confidence.)

   • The fear is something you need to talk through with another individual. (Honest communication fosters peace, harmony, and connection.)

6. Do the work, Mama. And remember, you are a fear-slaying warrior woman.

SECOND TRIMESTER

THE
GOLDEN AGE

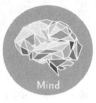

CHAPTER SEVEN

CREATING THE BIRTH SANCTUARY

JUST BREATHE: *Sitting straight, release any confusion in your mind by inhaling deeply through your nose, then pursing your lips and doing a strong exhale, making a "whoosh" sound. Do this ten times, with the intention that your mind will be clear and ready to make decisions after the final whoosh.*

The environment you birth in can make the difference between being pushed over the edge into a valley of orgasms and being pushed into a monologue of profanity. Your birth sanctuary will affect the energy surrounding your birthing experience and should be selected and set up with care. The environment in a hospital is vastly different from the environment in your home, yet both options offer elements that can be crucial to the creation of your peaceful birth, depending on your needs and preferences.

This chapter asks you to examine your birthing environment needs. If a hospital is where you intuitively believe you will be most comfortable, I encourage you to follow that instinct. If you have a strong urge to birth in your home, I'll support you in learning how to safely bring that desire to fruition. You'll learn to adapt your selection of care providers to work in harmony with your choice of birthing place, and with these elements decided upon, you can begin to add other elements of support (like hiring a birth doula).

Select the Sanctuary

Before getting nitty and gritty with your birth environment needs, let's pour the foundation. Where do you want to birth? In a hospital, birth center, or at home? Because each birthing facility is unique, I recommend touring the hospitals and birth centers in your area that would be feasible options for you. Ask questions, make sure you see all the areas you would be spending time in, meet the staff, and do whatever else you need to do to get a full sense of what it would be like to birth there. Let out a few howls to see how the acoustics are.

If you're considering a home birth, do a walk-through of your rooms, asking your Self if she would feel safe and relaxed birthing there. Is there a particular room you would like to birth in? Is there a separate area for your birth tribe to convene in when you want more privacy? Is there outside noise (maybe ongoing construction) that would impede your ability to get into that valley of orgasms? Do you have children or animals whose need for care would distract you from birthing? Do you *want* to birth at home?

Once you've narrowed down your choices, continue to examine the birth must-haves that make you most comfortable. Here are a few questions to spark the inquiry process.

- Will you feel more comfortable with hospital support close by? Or will a medical atmosphere cause you anxiety?
- Do you feel safest in your home?
- Do you have a medical condition that would make it risky for you to deliver at home, or in a birth center?
- Are you concerned you'll be tempted to request medical intervention if you're at the hospital? Do you feel this intervention would prevent you from having the unique birth you're hoping for? (It's easier to have a shot of Pitocin, with an epidural chaser, when you're sitting right there at the bar.)
- Do you *love* your medical care provider, and are you certain you want them to attend your birth? At which locations will they be able to attend your birth?
- What options does your health insurance cover?
- Where would you like to receive your prenatal care?

- Would you like a water birth? (Water births are more common in birth centers or home births.)
- How long does it take you to drive to the birth location in traffic? Are you comfortable with that commute?
- Are you at risk for preterm labor? If so, you may want to find a hospital with an excellent neonatal intensive care unit (NICU).
- If you're considering a hospital, what is their cesarean birth rate? If you would like to avoid a C-section, consider finding a hospital that is more inclined to support vaginal births.
- For a hospital birth, what is the nurse-to-patient ratio?
- What is the center's postpartum care protocol? Do they support immediate skin-to-skin time? Do they allow Baby to stay with Mom at all times (if both Mom and Baby are healthy)? How long is the typical stay after a birth?
- If you're considering a birth center, is it accredited by the Commission for the Accreditation of Birth Centers? How often do they transfer to a hospital? What professionals do they have on staff, or utilize as consultants?

If you live in a more rural area, your options may be limited. In this case, know you can infuse the energy you desire into any location — even if it's not your first choice   with the right people and key elements.

Hospitals Don't Have to Be Cold and Clinical

With the exception of open flames, you can pretty much bring whatever you like to a hospital birth to set the mood. You have the power to adjust lighting, temperature, sounds (blast those Ayurvedic chants or some AC/DC through your portable speaker), and smells. And you can shift other factors, such as people in the space (by requesting a different nurse, or maybe asking your freaked-out sister to leave), setting up a table full of crystals (seen it, and been asked to do it), having nonessential medical equipment removed from your room, changing the linens, and pretty much every other environmental element you would like to shift.

Having a list of birth preferences is another integral aspect of ensuring that your hospital birth sticks as close to your desires as possible. Hiring a doula (discussed further in this chapter) can also add a heightened level of support to any type of birth, but especially in the hospital, where doctors and nurses are rarely able to provide much support beyond the medical aspects of your care.

Birth Centers

Birth centers are a happy medium for women who aren't comfortable birthing at home but who get a case of the heebie-jeebies in a hospital. Birth centers are often located near a hospital and offer many of the comforts of home, like a cozy bed, Jacuzzi tub, soft lighting, comfortable couches and chairs, privacy, and quiet (unless you feel like hollering). Many midwives who practice out of a birth center perform all prenatal checks in this location, allowing you to become familiar with the environment before The Day.

Birthing centers often give Mom a greater sense of empowerment, because they won't expect her to go through routine medical protocol, often performed at hospitals, such as the administration of an IV or numerous vaginal exams. (But please remember you have the right to turn down any routine medical interventions during a hospital birth.) This environment promotes your ability to have a drug-free birth, if that's the option you feel best with, as your care providers will be trained to guide you into a more relaxed state with techniques such as massage, water, encouraging words, optimal birthing positions, and more.

You'll be a candidate for a birth center delivery only if you are having a "low-risk" pregnancy. While many birth centers have "light" medical equipment (e.g., IVs, oxygen, and certain medications like antibiotics and some analgesics), they do not provide medical induction, epidurals, or cesarean births, and they often do less monitoring and fewer vaginal exams. If you would like more "hands-on" medical attention, I recommend opting for a hospital birth.

Packing List for the Hospital or Birth Center

Here are a few things to consider as you're packing your hospital or birth center bag:

- What are the bare necessities I need? (Avoid overwhelm by packing only the essentials.)
- Do I love this item? (Consider this especially for focal point items or other extras that will serve more as decoration.)
- Will I use this item?
- How will I feel if I lose this item? (A lot of shuffling happens during birth; if you'll be devastated if the item gets lost in the flux of birth, leave it at home.)
- How conducive to organization is my luggage? (Choose a bag with various compartments so you can organize your belongings in categories, making it easier to quickly retrieve an item.)

For Mom

- Birth folder: ID, insurance card, one- or two-page document listing your birth preferences, and other needed paperwork
- Phone and charger
- Slip-on shoes (All kinds of gooey goodness will have graced the floors.)
- Two bathrobes and/or nightgowns: one for birth, one for after
- Loose and comfortable clothing (Two or three outfits; no skinny jeans — the snug waistband will just laugh at you.)
- High-waisted black "granny panties" to hide the postpartum bloodstains that will inevitably escape the boundaries of your thick pad)
- Toiletries (dental, hair, skin, and eyes)
- Light snacks (protein!) and electrolyte-rich fluid (coconut water!)
- A knowingness that *you can and will* do this!

For Birth Companion

- Phone, charger, and a clear smartphone photo album to fill with the most photos ever taken in a forty-eight-hour period
- Loose and comfortable clothing (two or three outfits)
- Toiletries (dental, hair, skin, and eyes)
- Light snacks
- Cash for vending machine

- Confidence, deep breaths, and love
- The pregnant lady!

For Baby

- Two or three outfits
- Blanket (This is for the car ride only — you don't want it to get lost in the laundry at the birth center or hospital.)
- Car seat already installed in car
- Diapers and wipes, if you have a specific brand you would like to use
- Bottles and formula if you will not be breastfeeding

Extras

- Birth ball
- Essential oils and electronic diffuser (Consider lavender, peppermint, or any other favorites. A few drops of peppermint oil in the toilet bowl will help you pee!)
- Pillow (There's a special place in Lame Town reserved for hospital pillows.)
- Birthing jewelry (Nothing expensive!)
- Birthing token (crystals, mandala, baby bamboo plant, stuffed unicorn?)
- Whatever makes you smile

Even if you're not having a home birth, I recommend reading through the following sections, which offer tips that could be beneficial in any birth location.

What You Need for a Home Birth

You don't need to be a placenta-stir-frying, dreadlock-rocking, screen-free maven to get blissed out with a home birth. (And if you are one of these mavens, you don't *have* to have a home birth! Birth where you want, Girl!). You may feel really safe and happy in your own home, which makes it a natural option for birth. If this is the space you've selected, move through the following considerations and suggestions to give yourself the best chance at having a harmonious home birth.

Care Provider

Most obstetricians will not, or cannot, attend a home birth, so go ahead and cross them off your list. However, most midwives and many naturopathic physicians and family practitioners are *so* up to get down with a home birth.

Word of mouth is the most powerful advertisement. Ask your already-done-it home-birthing mama friends which care provider they used. Did your friend like this person? Did they respect Mama's wishes? Did they put Mama at ease? Would your friend use them again? Compile a list of the best contenders and meet them. Sit down face to face and ask them every question your pregnant brain can remember. (Or bring a cheat sheet. Yeah, bring a cheat sheet.)

With your birth companion present, interview the candidates, giving them a full breakdown of the type of birth you would like to have so they can tell you if they think they'd be a good fit for you. Then, give yourself some time to ruminate on your options. Who had that special je ne sais quoi? Who had the best hair? Or stick to the basics: Who did you like best and was most willing to fully support your birthing desires?

Once you've made your selection, have another meet-up with your care provider to go over your birth preferences, making a plan for next steps. Many medical care providers for home births work with a specific hospital and obstetrician, in case of emergencies. Ask to meet with this OBGYN, and tour the hospital so you're familiar with the individual and alternative birthing environment should their services be needed. Having this "just in case" OBGYN can help soothe many latent fears and fend off Murphy's Law.

Doula

Once I told someone I was a doula and their response was, "So, are you a witch? Do you know potions?" The person was seven, but still, this word confuses people.

A doula supplies physiological and psychological support during and after birth. They act as your right-hand woman, or man, helping to make your experience happy and stress free. Doulas are not medically trained, and they do not administer medicine or perform clinical or medical tasks, but their presence can still be highly beneficial to Mom, Baby, and Birth

Companion. Doulas do not replace the birthing companion; they just offer additional support.

Birth doulas are specifically trained to support you during pregnancy and childbirth, usually being on-call for two weeks before and after your due date. Postpartum doulas support Mom and Baby after birth, often coming to the home for a couple hours a few days each week following the birth. Postpartum doulas often provide emotional support and breastfeeding assistance, perform household chores, and offer any other (nonmedical) support the family needs.

Here are a few of the many ways a birth doula can be of service:

- Provides continuous emotional support: helping to reduce fears and anxieties, bolstering confidence and a sense of empowerment
- Provides information in regard to birthing terminology, etc. (They do not give medical advice.)
- Offers pregnancy and birthing massage
- Provides a buffer in "harsher" birthing environments
- Maximizes the bonding between Mom and Birth Companion
- Offers aromatherapy
- Offers acupressure
- Provides visualization prompts
- Provides breathing technique prompts
- Provides assistance with various relaxation techniques, such as hypnotherapy
- Advocates for Mom and Birthing Companion in regard to birthing preferences
- Sets up birthing tub
- Assists with various birthing positions
- Serves as photographer and videographer
- Offers breastfeeding support
- Provides infant care training
- Prepares food
- Offers postpartum cleanup

When selecting a birth doula, or a postpartum doula, ask for referrals from local moms. Meet with a few before hiring; you want to ensure that you both think the relationship would be a good fit. Keep in mind that some doulas specialize in certain areas, such as massage or hypnotherapy, and they occasionally have higher rates because of this additional training. Choose the doula you and your birth companion feel great about!

IS A BIRTH DOULA WORTH IT?

Here are a few fun stats found in the *Cochrane Reviews* to confirm the wisdom of hiring a birth doula (the authors merged the results of twenty-two trials that included more than fifteen thousand women):

- Women who received continuous support during birth were more likely to have a spontaneous vaginal birth and were less likely to have medical interventions such as epidurals, forceps-assisted birth, induction medication, and cesarean sections.
- The women who received this support had labors that were about forty minutes shorter, on average, than the deliveries of women without continuous support.
- These babies were more likely to have higher Apgar scores (a quick test done on babies a few minutes after birth to summarize their health) than babies whose mamas did not have continuous support.
- When a doula was the individual providing the continuous support, the following results were found:
  - o 31 percent decrease in the use of synthetic oxytocin (Pitocin)
  - o 28 percent decrease in the likelihood of a C-section
  - o 12 percent increase in chance of spontaneous vaginal birth
  - o 9 percent decrease in use of pain medication
  - o 14 percent decrease in chance of infant being admitted to the NICU
  - o 34 percent decrease in chance of the mother being dissatisfied with her birth experience

Clearly, a doula is worth the moola.

Selecting a Special Space for Your Home Birth

Let's get mystical for a minute. Are your emotions tweaked when you walk into some spaces? Do you tap into the vibe those areas are throwing your way? Even if you're not consciously aware of these shifts, you're affected by the energy in different spaces. This energy will affect your birth. If you're having a home birth, you're in the unique position of having multiple rooms to choose from.

Selecting a space ahead of time is ideal, as it helps you contain the enormity of birth. Waiting until you're struck with surges to figure out where to "do the birth" can be overwhelming. Having a space set up for your birth needs ahead of time, filling that space with peaceful energy through meditation, and removing any chaotic energy (and stainable items) via decluttering and cleaning will give you an anchor when labor begins. You won't be wondering where you need to be; you'll go straight to your predetermined space and start doing the dang thang.

When selecting your baby-birthing zone, first meander through your home. Spend a few moments in each room, meditating on the areas where you feel best. Once you've determined your favorite areas, ask yourself the following questions, ultimately selecting the space that meets a majority of your criteria:

• Is there enough room for a birthing tub? Is there an adjoining bathroom with a built-in tub? Is this area close to a water source, for easy tub filling?

• Is there enough space for a birth ball? Is there a gliding or rocking chair that can support me in an upright position, while still allowing me the pleasure of movement?

• Will this area be comfortable for my birthing tribe? Are there chairs and couches for them to sit on? Or, will I want them to hang in another room and enter my birth space only when I request their assistance?

• Will this room facilitate an easy transition from birthing to postpartum care? Do I want to use this space for postpartum bonding, or do I want to move to another room?

• How close is the bathroom? (You may not be up for a long shuffle to the b-room during birth.)

• Is the lighting adjustable? Can I close the curtains to create a darker environment? Are there various lamps at different levels that can be

adjusted to suit my needs during labor? (Lighting has a powerful effect on the energy in a space, and low lighting can help your shy vagina open up.)
- Where do I *feel* best? Where does my intuition want to birth?

Ideally, you will have one space that accommodates all your desires, so you won't have to hoof it to different rooms while you're allowing a human to emerge from your vagina.

To Tub, Or Not to Tub?

Laboring in water is a trendy-train worth hopping on. Utilizing a tub during labor alleviates muscle tension, blurs the naked body (not that you need to hide those sexy curves!), contains all that juicy birth fluid, creates a type of weightless effect, and aids in the process of opening.

You have numerous tub options — an inflatable kiddie pool, a classic porcelain tub, or a birthing-specific tub. If you plan on spending a majority of your labor in water I would recommend renting a birthing tub. Most come equipped with a built-in padded seat for Mom, offer disposable liners, come in various sizes, and have adjustable height capabilities, proper stability, and more.

If you're into those perks, acquire a birthing tub a month or so before your Guess Due Time and do a test run by filling the tub with air and sitting in it to ensure there are no leaks; you'll have enough surprises on the day of delivery. If you already have a kiddo, let them play around in the waterless tub with you, to build their excitement about Baby's arrival.

If you would like your baby to actually be born in the water, consult with your care provider as to what sanitation measures need to be taken to ensure a healthy aqueous Earth entry for Baby.

Supplies

Many birth professionals come with a few of their own goodies, but they will rely on you to provide a majority of the birthing supplies. Here is a common list of what you'll need to have stored in the birth space, ideally a month before your care provider says your baby *may* come out. Your care provider will likely provide you with a list as well.

- **Birth ball:** Helps release pressure from the pelvic area, can easily be rinsed off, facilitates rhythmic motions, provides gentle pregnancy and postnatal exercise opportunities, and offers your eventual toddler a giant object to push around. You can also purchase a birth ball in your chosen birthing color, giving you a "too big to miss" focal point during labor.
- **Sanitized sheets, towels, and receiving blankets:** The linens you'll want to use for your birth will likely be the old dusty ones sitting in the dark recesses of your hall closet. Give them a ride in the washing machine. Wash two pairs of old sheets, four old full-size towels, four to six washcloths, and two receiving blankets. To prevent redustification, store your clean linens in a clear sealed container.

  When it's time, have your birth companion put a fresh set of "normal" sheets on your bed, a plastic sheet on top, and a pair of birth sheets on top of that. When baby is out, and you're ready to cozy up in some unsoiled sheets, strip off the amniotic fluid sheets and plastic sheet, and wham-bam-thank-you-man: fresh bed!
- **Birth kit:** Some genius thought up the idea of creating ready-to-go home birthing kits for purchase! Order one. These kits often include typical nonmedical birthing and postpartum supplies you would find at most birthing centers or hospitals. Ask your care provider if there is a particular birthing kit they can recommend for purchase.
- **Essential oils and diffuser:** Birthing spaces can take on weird odors when you're in the thick of it. Set up an electronic essential oil diffuser and select your favorite oils. Lavender is the classic choice for relaxation, and peppermint for stimulation, but have any of your other favorites on hand as well.
- **Perineal massage oil:** Make sure this is an oil with only one ingredient (e.g., coconut or jojoba oil).
- **Snacks:** Your favorite forms of protein.
- **Coconut water:** Electrolytes are really helpful to your birthing efforts.
- **Birthing jewelry:** Optional. If you have a piece of jewelry (one that's not expensive and can get wet without complaint) that evokes a happy or centered energy in you, go ahead and wear it.

- **Focal point:** Use the suggestions below to select one or more focal points you can use during birth.

Focal Point

As peaceful as staring at a blank wall, black screen, or napping birthing companion might be, I recommend choosing a calming focal point to focus on during birth. Select one or two of the feng shui symbols below, or any other image, sculpture, fountain, plant, or random item that fills you with good vibrations, then place it in an easy-to-view location. If you end up wanting to close your eyes and travel within, this focal point will serve as inspiration for the images floating through your mind.

Here are a few feng shui favorites:

- **Phoenix** symbolizes strength, resilience, and transformation.
- **Crane** promotes the energy of a long, peaceful, and noble life.
- **Peacock** invites protection and awareness into your life.
- **Magpie** is associated with "nesting" and children.
- **Fruit** promotes longevity, prosperity, and fertility.
- **Mystic knot** symbolizes the Buddhist belief in endless reincarnation.
- **Buddha** — his peace and joy are infectious!

The following colors can also evoke helpful energy during birth:

- **Earth hues (yellows and beige):** These colors will ground and center you, serving as a reminder that you are experiencing a natural process that is not to be feared.
- **Water hues (blue and black):** Just as actual water will bring comfort during birth, the blue and black feng shui water element colors will promote a calm and easy energy in your environment.

Home Birth Checklist

- Select your care providers and additional support (midwife? birth doula? backup OB?).
- Select the birthing space.
- Order birthing tub, hose, and shower hose adapter (optional).
- Assemble birth supplies: birth ball, sanitized sheets, plastic bottom

sheet, towels, receiving blankets, premade birth kit (order online), essential oils and diffuser, perineal massage oil, birthing jewelry, and focal point.

Birth Space To-Do List: Five Weeks before Guess Due Time

- Declutter.
- Have *someone else* readjust furniture (if needed).
- Remove "stainables."
- Gather and store the supplies.
- Set up a focal point and other extra supplies.

First Sign of Labor To-Do List

This list is for the birth companion; all you need to do when you go into labor is breathe, and do whatever else you feel like.

- Take a deep breath.
- See if Mom wants to rest, bathe, eat, or whatever.
- Call care provider. (Ask your care provider when they want you to call. Most say "when surges are four to five minutes apart" or "when surges are so strong Mom can't talk through them.")
- Call doula.
- *Do not* call family until you 100 percent know this is happening.
- (For nonhome birth) Make sure bag is ready to go and ensure house and any animals or children are set before departure.
- (For home birth) Prep bed: put regular sheets on, then plastic sheet, then freshly washed birth sheets on top.
- (For home birth) Set up birthing tub and make any last-minute adjustments to birth room.

From Her Heart to Yours

I had an unintentional home birth in a room I had subconsciously prepared for birth.

I was turned away at the hospital when I presented at only 3 cm. I cried on the car ride home, then climbed into my tub and listened to birth affirmations on repeat. In the preceding month, I had been compelled to fill this bathroom with my favorite candles, a sheepskin rug, blackout curtains, and a charging station for my portable stereo. These elements allowed me to slip deeply into birth and dissociate from everything happening around me.

While I was "out," my doula had called over a midwife, and I was brought back with a gentle hand on my shoulder and a voice asking if she could "check me." I agreed then heard I was "at a nine." We (myself, doula, midwife, husband, and OB) made the collective decision to switch to a home birth, and I birthed my baby on a daybed in the bathroom an hour later. I had my optimal birth in an optimal space, even though its unfolding was totally insane.

— *R. W., Santa Cruz, California*

RIDDLE: If you'll be birthing at home or at a birth center, I'm the care provider you should have on call in case you need any medical interventions. I like to hang out at the hospital, specifically the OR. What is the five-letter acronym used to describe what type of care provider I am?

Go to **YourSereneLife.wordpress.com/chapter-seven** and use the five-letter riddle answer as your offer code to download the relaxation recording for this chapter.

CALL TO PLEASURE

- Print out (or earmark) any of the checklists in this chapter that apply to you, edit them as needed for your unique needs, then follow them when the time comes.

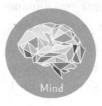

CHAPTER EIGHT

BIRTH PREFERENCES
Planning for Positivity

JUST BREATHE: *Allow each deep inhalation to draw out your intuition from the recesses of your subconscious mind, then with each exhalation allow the voice of your intuition to flow out of you. Do this as you contemplate each birth preference, allowing your intuition to write your birth plan.*

Acontractor uses blueprints to build a house. Sure, those plans change, maybe hundreds of times, before the house is complete, but it would be a total disaster without those initial plans. Don't build your child's birth without a set of plans. (And remember, if you don't have a clear vision for your birth, someone else will.)

As we weave through this chapter, I will help you get clear about your birthing blueprint (your preferences) and, importantly, help you get comfortable with possible changes to these desires. This well-thought-out list is the guide that will rally your birthing village, inform your birthing experience, and empower you to achieve your optimal birth, even if it veers far from certain aspects of the original draft. You will finish this chapter with a powerful one- or two-page document that clearly gives voice to your preferences and sets you up for greater satisfaction when you go through labor and delivery. This exercise is utterly empowering and, paradoxically, prepares you to ride the rapids of unpredictability that your birthing experience may bring.

You'll learn to set a Tone of Unity, ensuring that all participants in your birth know you're in it together and that you all want the same outcome of healthy Mom and Baby. We'll cover your preferences during the onset of labor and admission to your birthing space (hospital, birth center, home), desires for the opening and thinning phase of birth, your baby's descent, the birth, and your requests for the treatment of your baby after she is born.

Tone of Unity

Before you present your preferences to your birth tribe, set a tone of unity. You're not going into battle, so there's no need to pull rank. Hold on to the knowing that your birthing tribe wants you to have a beautiful and healthy birth. Preface your presentation of the preferences with a nonconfrontational "pep talk," reminding everyone that you want to go into birth with a harmonious tribe, committed to working together without individuals pushing their own ideas for how your birth "should be." Remind them that these are preferences, not demands, and you will do whatever is needed should the health of your baby or your Self be at risk. Set the intention with them that these preferences are a foundation to build your optimal birth upon.

Around this time, you may still be hit with ideas from your supporters about what decisions you should make. Those differing ideas are fine, and really they're none of your business. *Your* business is to ensure everyone understands that the preferences you're presenting are what you feel are right for your unique experience. Others don't have to agree that your desires are "right" — they just need to agree to fully support you in them. If they inform you that they can't support you, thank them for their honesty and find someone who can.

It's unlikely you'll experience a flat-out refusal of support, but you may encounter initial resistance. Meet any resistance with discussion, not anger. If the resistance is coming from your care provider, ask them questions about why they're hesitant about supporting you in a certain preference. Does their concern stem from your medical history? Hospital policy? Their own beliefs? Continue the discussion until you understand their position and can make an informed decision about whether you're going to keep the preference, take it out (without any resistance on your end), or find a different supporter (which is *absolutely* your prerogative).

If you're nervous about presenting your preferences to your care provider, which is very natural, write out a script to help you clarify your thoughts before speaking them.

Sampler Platter of Preferences

I'm now going to serve up many potential birth preferences for you. It's unlikely you will need to include all of them in your final list — many hospitals have begun shifting their protocols to include a majority of the preferences I'm going to cover (yay!). If you're having a hospital birth, I recommend taking the tour and asking as many questions as you can before printing out your final preferences.

If there are any preferences you feel indifferent about, don't include them — we want the desires you feel strongly about to stand out. If you prefer options I don't include, add them! There are no silly preferences, as long as they're important to you. One of my clients was adamant that everyone in her birth space wear seafoam green; it was her birth color and she used it to place her Self in a "soothing sea" mind-set. That was in her birth preferences.

Birth preferences are not just for natural births. If you plan to have an epidural, or any other medical assistance during birth, it will serve you to write up a plan for how you would like that experience (ideally) to flow. I have also included a "Cesarean Birth Preferences" section at the end of this chapter. From the preferences listed below, select those that you feel apply to the type of birth you believe is best for your individual needs.

To download the complete list of preferences, go to the following link: YourSereneLife.wordpress.com/birth-preferences.

Onset of Labor

Here are some preferences for the period after initial onset of labor.

- **To keep doing what I'm doing until I am intuitively ready to go to my birthing location:**
  - Go to sleep
  - Eat
  - Walk around

o Watch a movie
o Take a bath

If you feel comfortable at home, in the movie theater, restaurant, putt-putt golf course, or wherever you may be when labor begins, you may prefer to stay there. Unless there is a special circumstance requiring that you receive support from a care provider at the first sign of labor, this preference will help you plan to keep doing what you feel like doing until your intuition tells you to call in additional support.

One mama I worked with was about to start a dinner party at her home when she was kicked with the first signs of labor. She felt calm and comfortable and chose to continue on with the gathering. She had contractions throughout the dinner, but was so distracted by her company she barely noticed. Her baby was born at home shortly after the party ended.

This is *your* birth — do whatever *you* feel like!

Admission

These preferences can be chosen for admission to your birth facility.

- **To be free to go home if my cervix has not progressed to 4–6 cm dilation:** Think about what you'd prefer to do if you're not "adequately" dilated when you enter the birthing location. You may want to hug the nurse or midwife if she tells you you're not far enough along and should go home, or you may want to convince them to let you stay because you feel more comfortable at the hospital or birth center. Maybe you have no idea what your preference is, and that's okay. If you select this preference, know that you can change your mind in the moment, if that's where your intuition is leaning.

- **To decline IV:** Here are some common reasons it is protocol in many hospitals to administer a hep-lock (an IV that is capped off for potential later use) when Mom is admitted to hospital: to deliver fluids, administer any needed antibiotics or requested pain medications, or to have Mom "ready to go" in the case of an emergency cesarean birth. If you have no special circumstances and feel a hep-lock would distract you from relaxing, discuss your options with your care provider and add this preference to your final list. If an IV doesn't bother you and you feel you'd be more comfortable having it administered, skip this preference.

- **To have only occasional monitoring, unless there is a medical situation that requires otherwise:** In the absence of a special circumstance that would require you to be constantly monitored, you may request to have the sensors (that monitor baby's heart rate and your uterine contractions) removed in between readings. It's difficult to do laps in the hall, soak in warm water, or belly dance when you have monitor-appendages.

- **To discuss "comfort" rather than "pain" levels:** Your body is a robot that takes orders from your mind. When the mind is asked how much pain you're in, the body responds with the creation of pain so you can answer the question. With this preference you delete the word *pain* from your birthing vocabulary, and ask your supporters to do the same. Request that they ask you how much *comfort* you're in instead. You may scream "None!" at them, but at least you're not being injected with the term *pain*. Or, your body may respond with enhanced comfort. Send your body blissful messages, and you will have a more blissful birth.

- **To not be shown the Pain Scale:** Have you seen that graphic in a doctor's office of cartoon faces ranging from "smiley" to "my life is over!"? That sign is the visual version of the word *pain*. You may ask for the graphic to be removed or covered up with a photo of a *smiling* baby.

- **To be free to adjust the birthing environment by turning on music, lowering lighting, and making any other desired changes:** You're paying good money to rent a room in a birthing facility — it is your right to adjust the environment until it suits your needs. The factors in your birth space affecting your five senses will have a powerful impact on how your birth progresses. For example, harsh overhead lighting and uncomfortable temperatures will put you in the mind-set of a caged reptile too anxious to birth. Preplan how your birth companion will modify the room (such as by adjusting the thermostat, plugging in an essential oil diffuser, closing the blinds, turning on a lamp, putting on some Enya, doing a séance to ward off evil spirits — whatever you like), and have them apply the modifications as soon as possible.

Opening and Thinning

Here are some preferences you may choose for the opening and thinning phases of labor.

- **To be free to move and position myself in whatever way feels most comfortable:** A well of comfort is available to you in the empty spaces in your birth room. You can claim that comfort by indicating on your birth preferences your desire to move into whatever position calls to you if you begin to feel trapped in pain or stagnant energy (which is often caused by holding your breath). Practice the birthing positions offered on page 192 so your body will organically know where to take you when the time comes.

- **To have limited vaginal exams, and only with permission:** Something going up your vagina can be very uncomfortable when you're focusing on having something come out of your vagina. Vaginal exams, used to determine how dilated and effaced your cervix is, can pull you out of your birthing rhythm. You may go through moments where you desperately want to know how far along you are; in that case, get that vaginal exam. If you would rather not, but people are saying you should, you may simply decline (unless there is a medical situation that requires a vaginal exam). Just to be sure everyone is on the same page, you can plan for this eventuality by adding this item to your birth preferences.

  Here's another thing to consider: If your water has already released and you're not in active labor, it may serve you to decline all vaginal exams. Bacteria cannot enter the inner world of your vagina and uterus unless they are introduced. A vaginal exam could introduce that bacteria, leaving you vulnerable to infection. Discuss these options and risks with your care provider.

- **To labor in tub (if available) or shower:** Soaking in warm water, or having water rain down on you, can flip your birthing experience from "Give me that flippin' epidural!" to "Wow, okay, I can do this!" If this sounds good to you and your care provider gives the go-ahead, add this item to your birth preferences. Being immersed in water in the later stages of labor can potentially reduce the stress of labor and diminish the chance of fetal complications. A few other water birth bonuses: a potential increase in energy, enhanced freedom of movement, more efficient surges, improved circulation (more oxygen for Baby!), lower blood pressure, an increase in endorphin release (less pain!), and a more elastic perineum — 'nuff said.

- **To eat and drink:** The belief that it's unsafe to eat and drink during labor has had a shakedown. A study by the American Society of Anesthesiologists has shown that many women benefit from a light meal during labor. It just makes sense that keeping yourself fed and watered during the most physically demanding journey you'll likely ever experience is important — even crucial. Becoming dehydrated during labor can awaken an angry mob of birthing challenges, and getting too tuckered out from a lack of calories is a common precursor of unwanted medical induction methods. Eating a handful of nuts with a side of coconut water could stave off the scrub-clad waiter with a syringe full of synthetic oxytocin. Pack your favorite protein-rich snacks, a big metal water bottle (with a straw), and a few bottles of coconut water (high in electrolytes, which are needed for muscle contractions) in your birthing bag, and add this item to your birth preferences.

- **To go without medical intervention, unless there is a medical urgency:** If you've decided against medical interventions (totally optional!), add that to your preferences and remind your care providers about it — often. Nurses and doctors are used to situations where medical intervention is desired. They're not trying to bug you by offering interventions; they're just doing what they know. It's your job (or your birth companion's) to be very clear about what medical assistance you do and do *not* desire.

- **To have a complete explanation and discussion regarding any needed medical intervention:** If you are in a situation where intervention is needed, exercise your right to receive a full explanation of your options and to request the time to make an informed decision that you feel intuitively good with. (The exception, of course, would be the true emergency.)

- **To use natural methods to reposition Baby (*rebozo*, breathing, hypnosis, etc.):** The optimal position for your baby is head down (vertex) with the back of his head facing the front of your body. This position aids in a smooth descent. Medical care providers are (usually) mega-talented at discerning what position baby is in just by poking around on your belly. Think about whether you'd like the option to use natural methods if Baby needs to turn his head a bit to the right, or a smidge to the left. These might include a rebozo, a length of fabric you wrap around your belly when you're on all fours. Someone continuously shifts the rebozo in the direction Baby needs to turn. Other methods include deep breathing that will provide Baby the space to move into the optimal position (babies often naturally know where they need to go); self-hypnosis, where you breathe deeply while envisioning Baby moving into the ideal position; or assuming a "head down, butt up" position, where you get on all fours, then rest your head on your arms while leaving your booty up in the air.

- **To be patient if labor rests, and to have the space to use natural methods to reinduce labor (nipple stimulation, rest, food and water, bathroom, etc.):** It's common for your baby and body to ask for a break at some point during labor. If there is no medical urgency to "get things going" stat, you can indicate that you'd prefer to take the space and time to restart labor naturally. You can plan to have your partner stimulate your nipples (which helps to release oxytocin), take a nap (your body may be exhausted!), eat and drink while your body isn't going through all kinds of crazy motions, go to the bathroom (a full bladder can easily impede baby's downward progress), or do anything else that sounds nice to you.

Descent

These are some preferences you may choose for your baby's descent.

- **To be in whatever position I find most comfortable:** *Some* care providers still like to stick you flat on your back, feet up in stirrups, when Baby is making her final decent, even though this position is known to not do Mom any favors. If your labor is moving along, free of special circumstances, you should be able to assume any position *you* want to. Think about whether you'd like to be able to squat on the floor, for instance, or rest your tushy on a birthing stool, stand up and lean your head against your partner, lay sideways on the bed — you can do whatever you like. Who cares if your care providers aren't as comfortable? They're not the one's pushing a human out of their vagina. What's more, getting in the position you instinctually feel good in will likely speed up this final phase of labor and make it easier on you, especially if gravity is able to get in on the action.

- **To be free of loud prompts to push:** If you feel you'll want loud reminders to "PUSH!" then skip this preference — some people thrive in a cheerleader-esque environment. But if people yelling at you during one of the most intense moments of your life will just piss you off, highlight this preference. Instead, request that *one person* gently guide you through the process of pushing Baby out, supporting you in knowing how and when to breathe and bear down, and offering loving encouragement in between.

- **To be in a quiet room, able to breathe my baby down to emergence, pushing only when I feel ready:** Instead of holding your breath and pushing until some hemorrhoids pop out, you may want to plan to take in a powerful inhalation during each surge, then envision that oxygen being pushed down the back of your throat and down and out your vagina as you exhale. If this sounds like something that might work for you, add it to your birth preferences.

This breathing will gently nudge Baby down, open your perineum (as opposed to constricting it), provide you and Baby with ample oxygen (during a stage in labor when oxygen is often in limited supply), and conserve your energy. And, when you feel an *overwhelming* urge to push, go for it, Mama!

Emergence

These preferences focus on Baby's emergence.

- **To allow my baby to emerge free of assistance from medical care providers, unless assistance is medically necessary:** Forceps all up in ya ("just 'cause") are so not en vogue anymore. Your birth preferences can request that your care provider keep their hands to themselves unless it is medically necessary for them to assist. The one exception is a perineal oil massage. Many care providers rub natural oil around Mom's perineum as Baby is emerging to soften the opening and encourage Baby's smooth emergence. This is good.

- **To avoid suctioning of my baby's nose and mouth unless medically necessary:** Baby is constantly inhaling and exhaling amniotic fluid while chilling in utero. As he is birthed, his body releases chemicals to help his lungs push out the fluid. The pressure of your birth passage also helps to release the fluid. When Baby is out, his coughing and breathing should expel any fluid still hanging out. Having a plastic bulb shoved into your nose and mouth right after you passed through a tight passage into a brand-new world sounds kind of intense, right? Your preferences can indicate that your baby be spared from this assault, unless your care provider feels the suctioning is vital for his health.

- **To have my birth companion or mother receive Baby after her head and shoulders emerge:** The first touch Baby receives after birth is sacred. If it's possible for you or your partner to be the first hands that kiss Baby's skin after birth (and you both feel comfortable with that), remind your care provider of this preference so they can guide you as to when and how to receive Baby.

- **To allow my placenta to be birthed naturally:** Your placenta (that amazing organ you grew to support your baby's development) will be coming out behind your baby. This usually happens within thirty minutes after birth and requires you to continue having uterine surges. But you'll be so distracted by the human you built and birthed that you won't be very concerned with the residual surges. It's common for care providers to do some poking around on the abdomen to monitor the placenta's progress, and they mostly stay south of the pelvic region until it's certain the entire placenta has been birthed.

- **To receive a synthetic oxytocin (Pitocin) injection only if medically needed to prevent hemorrhage:** It's common practice in many birth facilities to give Mom an injection of synthetic oxytocin directly after birth to ensure that her surges are strong enough to birth the full placenta. (If a portion of the placenta is not birthed, you could be at risk for hemorrhaging and the care provider may need to scrape the uterus, which is just as fun as it sounds.) If the thought of a postbirth injection doesn't bother you, I say go ahead and receive the injection. If you think the poke will pull you out of your baby-bliss zone, discuss with your care provider the option of not receiving the injection.

For Baby

Here are some preferences you may choose for Baby's care after emergence.

- **To not have vernix wiped off:** According to the *American Journal of Obstetrics & Gynecology*, the vernix (a cheese-like coating on Baby's skin) contains antimicrobial proteins that help to protect Baby from Group B strep, *E. coli*, and other prenatal yucks that could cause disease. This skin coating also helps to moisturize and cleanse Baby's skin. Instead of wiping it off, you may opt to gently rub the vernix into Baby's skin as he's lying on your chest. In lieu of a bath, you may wipe him off with a soft washcloth after you've had a few hours to bond and establish breastfeeding. If all this sounds good, add it to your birth preferences to make sure someone doesn't accidentally give your baby the customary postbirth wipe-down.

- **To have my baby placed on my chest as soon as possible:** Your body teaches your baby how to survive in this world, enhancing her physical, emotional, and developmental health. As a teacher, your body has total superhero status. Being on your chest, skin-to-skin, helps Baby regulate her breathing, heart rate, blood pressure, and temperature. (Your breasts will adjust their temperature to manage Baby's temperature!) These skin-to-skin benefits are believed to have a hand (or breast) in the correlation Dr. Sears found between co-sleeping and lower rates of SIDS (sudden infant death syndrome). If immediate skin-to-skin contact after a vaginal birth is not already protocol at the facility you'll be birthing in, add this to your list of birth preferences.

- **To allow my cord to finish pulsating before clamping:** It was once believed that cutting the cord ASAP lowered Mom's chances of hemorrhaging; studies published in the *Cochrane Reviews* found this to be false: Mom's chances of hemorrhaging are neither heightened nor lessened by delayed cord clamping. Baby, however, greatly benefits from being allowed to remain attached to his original lifeline until the process of receiving all the iron- and hemoglobin-rich blood from the cord is complete. Hemoglobin is the protein in red blood cells that carries oxygen, and oxygen is good. An iron deficiency is not good and can cause potential growth and developmental delays. And it's not like your baby will be attached until preschool. The cord usually stops pulsating within a few minutes, and can then be snipped.

  In certain circumstances, delayed cord clamping can cause a bit of jaundice (slight yellowing of the skin), which can be treated with phototherapy (exposure to sunlight).

  Beyond the physical benefits, delayed cord clamping can provide a more gradual transition for both Mom and Baby, who are trying to integrate with their new reality. Because of the symbolic magnitude of this severing of physical ties, you may want to ask your birth companion if they feel comfortable doing the honors.

- **To delay application of prophylactic eye medication for one hour:** This eye salve, which comes in the form of drops, is meant to protect babies exposed to chlamydia or gonorrhea in the birth canal from developing ophthalmia neonatorum (ON), a type of pinkeye that has the potential to cause blindness. Even if the mother does not test positive for any STDs, it is common practice in most U.S. hospitals for all babies to receive these eye drops. Because the drops can cause Baby's already faulty eyesight to blur, it can be nice to delay the application (which needs to be given in the first twenty-four hours postbirth) so Baby can visually bond with you and your partner.

- **To have my baby with me and my companion at all times:** You are *everything* to your baby, and the feeling is likely mutual. Being separated, even for a few moments, can be very disorienting for both of you. If there is no medical reason for you and Baby to be apart, you may request that she be weighed, bathed, and given other needed assistance in the same room as you. The more time you're able to spend together, the greater your bonding and breastfeeding success will be.

You Rock

You might want to add to your birth preferences a quick thank-you for your supporters: *We thank you for supporting, respecting, and championing our optimal birth.*

At the end of your preferences, add a brief note of gratitude for your care providers, thanking them for doing everything in their power to follow your preferences as closely as possible and supporting you in your optimal birth, whatever that ends up looking like! A little bit of sugar for these hardworking folks goes a long way. Speaking of sugar…some women choose to add "Treat for Care Providers" to their packing list, so they can offer an edible piece of thanks to their supporters.

Remember that these preferences are just options, not commands for how you need to birth. Trust your instincts as you create this list, keeping what resonates with you, leaving out what doesn't, and adding new items you believe will support your birth journey.

Cesarean Birth Preferences

Many women feel strong resistance to cesarean birth because they believe they would have little control with this category of birth, which can drain their sense of empowerment. In the absence of an emergency, however, many hospitals are becoming more open to moms exercising their right to have a voice in how their cesarean birth unfolds. I've created these preferences with the courageous women I have supported in cesarean births. Their births were just as beautiful and powerful as many of the vaginal births I've witnessed.

In the case of a cesarean birth, you may request and of the following:

- **To have my arms free during the operation:** Being strapped down rarely feels good. You may request that your arms remain free so you can hold your baby as soon as possible after delivery.

- **To have skin-to-skin contact directly after my baby is born:** We've discussed the importance of skin-to-skin contact after birth. These benefits are even more crucial for a mom and baby who have traveled through a cesarean birth because they have not had the time to gently integrate into the emergence of new life, or to release the "feel good" hormones that build up during vaginal birth. Skin-to-skin contact in the first hour after birth (The Magical Hour) will stimulate the release of oxytocin (The Love and Bonding Hormone) in you and in Baby, playing a primary role in helping you "feel like a mother" and supporting the eventual act of breastfeeding.

- **To have the screen dropped the moment my baby is being born:** Seeing the moment of your baby's arrival is a powerful experience, especially for moms who cannot physically feel the emergence. If you feel comfortable having the screen between your upper and lower body lowered as Baby is pulled out of the womb, it could help you feel a deeper connection to your birth and baby.

- **To have medical staff refrain from personal conversations:** Talk about the anesthesiologist's date last weekend is unlikely to hold the sacred messages you want to be hearing as your baby is born. Request that all occupants of the operating room refrain from personal conversation, instead opting for encouraging words for you.
- **To have music or a recording of choice playing during the operation:** If listening to "Stayin' Alive" during your cesarean birth (true story) doesn't sound appealing to you, ask that your own music or relaxation recording be played during birth. Have these recordings easy to locate on your phone, and refrain from streaming music stations that play ads — a commercial for the latest horror movie is likely to be unappealing during birth.
- **To have nasal cannula instead of a face mask for oxygen:** If possible, ask that you be given oxygen via nasal cannula rather than a face mask if you feel the face mask will make you feel claustrophobic. It's also easier to kiss your baby when you don't have a hunk of plastic strapped to your face.

Go to the following link to download the Cesarean Birth Preferences template: YourSereneLife.wordpress.com/birth-preferences.

"Birth Plans Set You Up for Disappointment": I Call Bull!

If you tell someone you're working on your birth plan and they roll their eyes and say, "Birth plans set you up for disappointment," politely tell them "Hogwash!" and walk away.

Spending the time now to understand all your options and to marinate in your feelings about each one will allow you to enter your birthing space in a more relaxed and educated frame of mind. Some believe setting specific birth preferences is like trying to ensure that an unknown free-flowing energy will fit into a premade box; but the opposite is true. Creating your birthing preferences, informing and discussing the preferences with your birthing supporters (partner, mom, doula, care provider, tarot card reader, etc.), and practicing with your birth companion how you'll both advocate for your birthing preferences will set you free.

Birth preferences are similar to the preparation an actor does for a performance: They spend time examining every aspect of their character and going over their script so many times it becomes ingrained in their being. When it's time to perform, they let all the prep work go and allow it to naturally flow out of them. Putting in the prep time with your birthing preferences will allow decisions on The Day to flow easily from you and your companion, even if the decision is a tricky one. And unlike an actor, who needs to be "off-book" by the time of their performance, you'll have many copies of your script to pass out.

Belly Rubbing Meditation

While slathering "stretch mark preventing" coconut oil or shea butter onto your belly, close your eyes and place your hands on your belly, tapping lightly to bring your baby into the meditation. Begin rubbing the oil around in gentle circular movements, setting the intention that the energy being created by your movement is being transmitted to your baby, creating an intuitive connection between the two of you that will guide you while creating your birth preferences and moving through birth.

> **RIDDLE:** What hormone is released throughout birth and is known as The Love and Bonding Hormone?
>
> Go to **YourSereneLife.wordpress.com/chapter-eight** and use the one-word riddle answer as your offer code to download the relaxation recording for this chapter.

CALL TO PLEASURE

1. Do the Belly Rubbing Meditation daily to connect to your baby's intuition so he can have a say in the preferences.
2. Download the Birth Preferences Template from the following link: YourSereneLife.wordpress.com/birth-preferences.
3. Edit preferences to your liking; ignore what everyone claims you *should* want, and choose the preferences you actually resonate with.

4. Write the intro letter or script you will use to present the preferences to your birth supporters.
5. Print four copies of your birth preferences.
6. Give two copies to your medical care provider.
7. Keep two copies in your birth folder.

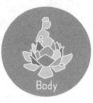

Body

CHAPTER NINE

NONTRADITIONAL PREGNANCY:
What If My Baby Doesn't Share My DNA, or My Womb?

Just Breathe: Breathe in the spirit of your baby by drawing on the power of the number one, which represents new beginnings, and the number two, which represents unity. Inhale slowly, repeating "one, two, one, two, one, two..." in your mind and heart until you can no longer inhale, then exhale, repeating the same number sequence. Let this exercise be a reminder that while you may not share DNA with your baby, or he might not be growing in your womb, you can still connect deeply to his spirit — forging a powerful bond before he's in your arms.

The urge to achieve physical immortality through procreation is an innate need in many humans, a need that is being shattered in our increasingly infertile culture. Now that egg donors, sperm donors, and gestational surrogates are a new fixture in the wheelhouse of pregnancy, many women are navigating an unexpected reality: the child in their womb does not share their own DNA, or the DNA of their partner, or their baby is growing in the uterus of a gestational surrogate. As you move into the second trimester, your belly bulge (or that of your surrogate) begins to grow and the baby's movements become noticeable — the baby now seems "real."

This is often when women with nontraditional pregnancies face a confusing turmoil of emotions.

When you received the positive pregnancy results, did you feel a wave of relief and elation swoop through you? Did you hear the cheer of "Yes! We've made it!" ring through your heart? I hope so! You deserve to revel in the fact that your efforts (and perhaps your hefty financial investment) created the spark of new life. But, now that your baby is deep into development, you're dunked into a fresh reservoir of "holy shifts."

I'm going to guide you through the process of integrating with this novel landscape of nontraditional baby making, exploring the strata of feelings, insecurities, overwhelming unknowns, shame, anxiety, anger, and onward you've likely been traveling through for quite some time. We'll also explore how to shift focus from "physical immortality" to "spiritual immortality."

Parents navigating the adoption process can also pull support from these ideas.

Your Baby Is Coming to You in the Way the Universe Intended

As confounding (and painful!) as it can be at times, the universe does not make mistakes. It is bringing your baby to you in the exact way she was meant to come. If your nontraditional pregnancy was caused by something you feel you did "wrong," I want to work with you to dissolve that. If everything had not aligned in the precise way it has thus far, the baby who is coming to you would not be in your reality. But she is! She is coming. The moment you first hold her in your arms and your eyes meet, you'll be filled with gratitude for all the challenges you went through to make this unique human a presence in your existence.

"Thank you, universe, for being so perfectly frustrating, perplexing, and all knowing!"

Even when you consciously believe that "everything happens for a reason," you still may experience a feeling of disconnection if your baby does not share the genetic makeup of both you and your partner, or share your womb. If the emotion of disconnection comes up, I want you to briefly close your eyes and explore the idea that we are all One — all derived from the same source — so that regardless of the physical nature of your pregnancy, you, your baby, and your partner already share a bond of Oneness that cannot be broken. When doubt about your journey flares up, return to the simple truth of Oneness. This return to a belief in Oneness can also awaken a hope that although "physical immortality" may not be an ingredient in your pregnancy, you're receiving the ultimate gift of achieving spiritual immortality by leaving an Imprint of Love on your baby's spirit — which is way cooler than a couple of strands of genetic instructions.

Let's explore the unique challenges mamas and papas face in the three primary categories of "untraditional" pregnancy.

Baby Conceived with Donor Egg

There is a big vat stewing with different reasons women may need to use an egg donor: advanced maternal age, genetic disease, poor egg quality, history of pregnancy failure, and much more. You may have spent exhaustive years trying to create a successful pregnancy with your own DNA, so it can be deeply disappointing when a viable pregnancy does not result. Moving through the grieving process and releasing your ideas about what your baby "should be" (e.g., possessing your own genetic code) can be very painful, but is crucial to your ability to fully bond with the baby who is coming to you.

Feel it. Surrender to that grief via crying, journaling, attending support groups, or anything else you feel will clear the space of regret within you so you can fill it with love for your baby, whose genetics may not be derived from your own but whose spirit chose *you* as his mother. Your baby is no less a part of the true nature of *you* than a baby who sprouted from your egg.

It is also common to feel an undercurrent, oftentimes subconscious, of resentment toward the partner who *was* able to contribute their DNA to the baby. Make sure you also work through this (very natural) sentiment, so you can journey into parenthood as a united team.

If you are carrying Baby in your womb, set the intent that you are still able to offer a big piece of your physical self to the development of your baby through the food and drink you consume, the love hormones and endorphins that pass through the placenta, and the sacred blend of breast milk you may eventually nourish him with. *You are the mama* of this baby, who came to you for a reason; fill the space you created through clearing your regret with profound gratitude for this knowing.

Baby Conceived with Donor Sperm

A father who is not able to provide his DNA to the baby also needs to clear away any regret. To ensure he's able to move into parenthood with an open heart, it's also vital for him to explore any impact this may have had on his ego. (The same may also be the case for a woman using an egg donor.) Many humans pride themselves on their DNA and the ability to pass it on to future generations; when this ability is stifled, it can cause the ego to take a beating. Many dads I've worked with who have used a sperm donor expressed feelings of "being less of a man," "being deflated by misconceptions about my body's ability," or "a morphing of self-image." These are beliefs that deserve to be honored and explored.

The idea that "I just need to love my baby and get over my insecurities" does a disservice to both parent and baby. Those insecurities and regrets come up for a reason, and they often offer tremendous opportunities for growth if the parent is able to acknowledge and explore them, whether through crying, journaling, open communication, exercise, therapy, or other "clearing" activities. These clearing activities usually lead to an organic release of these limiting "less than" misconceptions. And remember, Dad, Baby's spirit did not just choose Mom, he also chose *you*.

Baby Carried in Another Womb

Not being able to provide baby with her first home can be a deep blow for parents. The physical experience of pregnancy and childbirth is at the forefront of many women's dreams about their first steps into motherhood, and missing that rite of passage can cause an initial sense of disconnection from your baby. But the sense of disconnection doesn't need to last. Nurturing the mind, body, and spirit of the woman carrying your baby is the same as nurturing the mind, body, and spirit of your baby. Just because you can't be the one to directly offer this support doesn't mean you're not facilitating it, which is just as significant. Ensure that your gestational surrogate has a nurturing environment to live in, nutrient-rich, organic food to fill your baby with, emotional support to encourage the release of "feel good" hormones, uplifting and informative classes to prepare her for birth, and a hearty dose of your voice so she can share it with your baby (this can come in the form of frequent visits or voice recordings of you singing or talking gently to Baby).

In addition to the tangible acts you can take to support your developing baby and gestational surrogate, you can practice the following daily meditation to send loving energy to your baby, creating a spiritual connection before she's in your arms:

- Sit in a quiet and comfortable location and set your timer for eight minutes (you can increase your time as you're able).
- Close your eyes, place your hands on your heart, and envision a bright light of love entering the top of your head and flowing through your entire body until you sense that you are pulsating with this light.
- Sit in this light for a few moments, *feeling* what it's like to be immersed in the pure light of love.
- Now, envision your baby in your mind's eye. This image can be whatever you like — a vision of a baby, a ball of light, or anything else that symbolizes your baby.
- Imagine the light of love (which you have a limitless supply of!) pouring from your heart center and filling and surrounding your baby.
- Be present in this space of love with your baby. Smile, cry tears of love, give her blessings, sing to her — communicate with her in whatever form you're called to, even if it's just silence.
- When your timer chimes, blow Baby a kiss and tell her that you'll return to her tomorrow.

How to Explain the Pregnancy to Loved Ones

Many people are like, "IVF…what? Does that stand for Inverted Vaginal Fertilization?" (Someone once spoke those exact words to me.) While IVF (in vitro fertilization) is becoming more prevalent in our society, it is still a huge question mark for many people, in a scientific, ethical, and emotional sense. If you kept your journey through IVF private, it can be a shock for friends and family to be met with the news that...

"We're pregnant! And we're using another woman's eggs!"

Or...

"We're pregnant! And we're using another man's sperm!"

Or...

"We're pregnant! And we're using another woman's womb!"

While it can be tempting to keep this information private (which is completely your right), sharing the untraditional (and very special!) nature of your pregnancy can open up your network of support during a time that will likely be very emotional, and potentially challenging, for both you and your partner. Your emotional journey may be more intense than that of those who are traveling through a "traditional" pregnancy. You didn't just have sex and "wham-bam, hey there, fertilized egg!"; you had to fight for your ability to conceive. You had to become a total mama warrior, and that can be soul-deep exhausting. You deserve to have a robust group of loved ones lifting you up and supporting you in all aspects of this new phase of your journey.

If you choose to go ahead and spill the IVF beans, it may be necessary for you to educate your friends and family on the basics of IVF and to give them the *CliffsNotes* explanation of your need to take this route. If you feel judgment from someone that you do not feel can be worked through, consider removing that individual from your inner cluster of supporters; your journey doesn't need any negative noise.

Have these conversations when *you* intuitively feel good and ready — all in your own time, Mama.

How to Tell Your Child, When He's Older

Whether or not to tell a child conceived or grown through IVF is a hotly debated issue, and a decision you and your partner should deeply discuss and explore. Some key points in this discussion are whether or not the child will need this information to make future health decisions (e.g., if he was conceived using donor DNA), whether or not it is fair and psychologically healthy to keep this information from the child, and whether or not the child should be allowed to have access to the identity of their egg donor, sperm donor, or gestational surrogate. So tricky!

It is important for all humans to know if they are potentially at risk for certain health problems. This information can give them the chance to take precautionary measures to help prevent the onset of these health issues. For example, if an egg donor's mother had heart disease, the donor-conceived child would have an increased risk of heart disease. If the donor-conceived child was aware of this information, he could make sure to have regular checkups, eat a healthy diet, and exercise regularly. It is possible for families to learn the medical history of their donor without the donor's identity being revealed.

Humans also have a fundamental interest in knowing about their biological origins. It is natural for a child to want to know the basics of the genetic code he came from. If you decide to disclose the use of a donor to your child, you can give a physical description of the donor, such as eye color, hair color, body type, height, ethnicity, and so on without disclosing the donor's actual identity. A study of California parents, "Strategies for Disclosure: How Parents Approach Telling Their Children That They Were Conceived with Donor Gametes," found that most children who know they were donor-conceived are very well adjusted, and that it is best to have this talk with children as soon as they're old enough to understand.

Although some donor-conceived children and their parents might have the desire to meet their donor, it is not their choice alone. The donor must be comfortable and willing to meet the family. There are some cases where the donor legally agrees before donation to have his or her identity made known to the parents and any children conceived through the donation, but most donations are made anonymously.

The decision of whether or not to inform donor-conceived children of their biological origins is a big decision that should be well thought out. You will have your own opinion on what information you should disclose to your children, and you should follow your instincts. When you keep the well-being of your child at the forefront of your mind, you can't go wrong.

Similar emotional considerations should be taken in the case of a gestational surrogate. Although the child is unlikely to share DNA with the surrogate, they still spent a sacred period of time together during the child's gestation. You and your surrogate may feel it is best for the surrogate not to be a part of your child's life, but discussing what the surrogate was like, pregnancy-specific experiences she had during gestation, and a (nongraphic) retelling of the birth can help to round out your child's knowledge of how they came to be.

Prenatal Bonding Activities

Your baby's extraordinary conception, gestation, and birth are flush with op-portunities for mega-bonding. But because it can be confusing (and daunt-ing!) to travel into the uncharted land of bonding with a child who did not come to you in the way you initially expected, it will simplify your postpar-tum bonding efforts to begin this venture of the heart now, before the birth. Start with the following:

- **IVF-specific children's books:** There are lovely books made for chil-dren born from donor DNA or a gestational surrogate. Choose a few of your favorites and begin reading them to Baby while she's in the womb. If you're using a gestational surrogate, send a recording of you reading the books that she can play for Baby.
- **Love letters:** Write a letter to your baby each month, describing how you're feeling about meeting her, dreams you have for her fu-ture, exciting adventures you'll have, April Fools' pranks you can pull on your partner together, and anything else you feel compelled to write about. The intent is to get in a zone where you feel an intimate connection with your baby, even if you're not physically together. If you are physically together, you can read her the letters as you go. These can also be sweet mementos to give your child when she's older.
- **Talkies and still shots:** Don't be shy of that selfie stick! Who cares if your chin and neck have become one, or your feet have eaten your ankles — you're *pregnant*, and you're gosh darn beautiful! If you are using a surrogate, take photos and videos with her (if she's comfort-able with the idea) to fortify your connection to the gestation of your baby and to the Earth Angel who has chosen to be the initial vessel for your baby's life.
- **Childbirth preparation classes:** Learning about what you (or your surrogate) will journey through during childbirth will make your

baby seem more real. Having an unseen, moving human in your body can feel very abstract — even more so when that human is in another woman's body. If you feel any doubt that your baby is actually coming into your life, childbirth preparation classes will plant your heart firmly in your beautiful reality.

RIDDLE: What three-letter acronym represents the process of an egg and sperm becoming one — outside the woman's body?

Go to **YourSereneLife.wordpress.com/chapter-nine** and use the three-letter riddle answer as your offer code to download the relaxation recording for this chapter!

CALL TO PLEASURE

- Every day, spend five minutes meditating on the fact that your baby is coming to you in the exact way he is meant to.
- With your partner, write out a list of talking points you will hit on when sharing the news of your pregnancy with friends and family.
- With your partner, write out a list of talking points you will use when discussing the nature of your child's conception or gestation with him. Though you won't use this list for many years, it will help to clear any anxiety you feel about sharing this delicate information with your child.

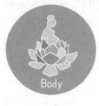

CHAPTER TEN

WATER, WATER, WATER — AND, OH YEAH, WATER!

JUST BREATHE: *Inhale slowly to a count of ten, envisioning your cells becoming porous and ready to receive the nourishing liquid you're about to ingest. As you exhale, imagine any negative energy that could be blocking your body's ability to take in the gift of water, and allow it to pour out of you. Now, take a big ole sip of water.*

Pregnancy will drive you straight to the bottle...of water. Because our bodies are about 76 percent water, and a baby at birth is around 94 percent water, we should all hail the goodness of this elixir of life, this essential base of everything happening in the body. And it's all happening, unless you're dehydrated. Embracing the mighty powers of water by making it your constant companion, preferably a companion housed in an easy-to-carry metal water bottle, will enrich your life with a sense of harmony and well-being you didn't even know you were missing. Beyond the physical treats water serves up, we'll also explore the spiritual aspects of water, water rituals, and water birthing in this chapter. I go beyond the common "drink eight glasses a day" advice to fill you with a reverence and renewed craving for this life source.

Elixir of Life

Not much happens without water — plants don't sprout, babies don't develop, hormonal pregnant women can't access their equilibrium (or regular bowel movements), and other fun events do not reach their full potential. Drink yo' water (or "wa-wu" in toddler-ese). A steady stream of clean water all up in you will wash away many of the unpleasant companions of pregnancy, such as ankles turned cankles, low levels of amniotic fluid (the liquid Baby floats in), urinary tract infections (UTIs), hemorrhoids, overheating, excessive weight gain, and anxiety. Water is also an essential element for Baby's development; it helps your body lap up the goodness you're feeding it and then transports those vitamins, minerals, and hormones to blood cells that are soaked up by the placenta, and then by your baby.

How to Get Enough of the Right Stuff

Huge metal water bottles were my jam during pregnancy — and I still rock that fluid-filled monstrosity with pride. Find yourself a large metal water bottle (preferably a forty-ouncer) and gulp it down regularly. A glass bottle with a protective rubber coating is another good option. Why not plastic? Even if a plastic product says "BPA-free" it could still house chemicals that could be unkind to your body. To further ensure your water is safe, have a faucet-mounted filter installed on your primary waterspout, or purchase a freestanding water-purifying pitcher.

If you get the aforementioned forty-ounce bottle, drink the first half of the bottle within thirty minutes after you wake up in the morning. This flushes out toxins that may have built up overnight, wakes up your metabolism and brain (the brain is 75 percent water), and helps regulate your appetite. Then set an hourly timer and spend five minutes slowly sipping your beverage every time it goes off. Add fresh lemon juice to your water to alkalinize your body, neutralizing any unhealthy acids.

Amp up your water intake (beyond one hundred ounces a day) before and after workouts, on hot days, if you're not urinating regularly, or if your pee is not close to colorless.

If taking in all this water begins to take on the same thrill level as eating saltine crackers, you can spice things up with coconut water, sparkling water, vegetable juice, almond milk, decaffeinated tea, or any other liquid that has not been imbued with alcohol, caffeine, or added sugar. You can also nosh on water-filled foods like watermelon, pears, or cantaloupe.

Infuse It with Love

Water is moody, sensitive to the energy it's exposed to — it will even change its composition to mirror that energy. This isn't *just* magic; it's magic that has married scientific observation. In 1994, Dr. Masaru Emoto and a team of researchers observed two sets of frozen water crystal specimens: one exposed to positive words, beautiful images, harmonious music, and blessings and the other exposed to negative words, images, and sounds. All of the samples exposed to the different forms of positive energy had transformed into beautiful symmetrical crystals, not one identical to any of the others. The samples exposed to negative messages, sounds, and images morphed into disfigured crystals.

Try one or all of the following suggestions to enrich your water with the energy you desire in your life:

- Write a positive word, like *love, healing, joy, gratitude, blessings,* or any other term that encompasses the vibes you would like to fill your whole being with, on a piece of paper and tape it to your water bottle. Set the intention that the spirit of that word transforms all the water that flows into the bottle.
- Before you take a sip of water, send gratitude to it for filling you with whatever you're in need of. As the water pours down your throat, feel yourself being filled with love, healing, joy, gratitude, patience, or whatever else you need.
- If you've chosen to have a natural birth, water can serve as your organic pain relief (working alongside your deep breathing and your endorphins). Each time you drink water during labor, envision it easing any discomfort you're experiencing by flushing it out and away. With every sip of water you become more and more comfortable.

Sacred Nature

Water covers approximately 71 percent of the Earth's surface and is the primary filler of our bodies. It is used to cleanse the bodies and shelters of Mother Nature, humans, and animals and has been known to draw a crowd because of its mass appeal.

But water is so much more than a life-sustaining workhorse. Water holds the memory of what it has passed through, water is forgiving, water is adaptable, water births community, water gives freely without asking for a drop in return, and water is a physical expression of love.

Spiritual leaders and traditions understand this sacred nature of water. Millions travel to shrines built around water sources believed to hold a connection to God. Many religions use water to christen, bless, initiate, and heal. Ancient cultures honored water as the origin of life, and it is the source of one of the only universal love affairs; its powers are so intoxicating it has brought warring nations to peace, in efforts to protect a shared water supply.

The most common way water is honored is through bathing. Wellsprings that are open for public bathing are the destination of many pilgrimages because it is believed that water is most sacred when it is first exposed to light and is still resonating with the richness of Earth's heart. A famous example is the Grotto of Massabielle in France, which has seventeen pools, all believed to possess healing properties.

If you don't have time to bathe in French holy water before your baby is born, here are a few ideas for creating your own rituals to connect with and honor water:

- **Gift offering:** Bring a gift (a rock, flower, leaf, or any other natural object you find special) to a source of water, give it a verbal blessing, and release it into the water source with the intention that the water will absorb your blessings.
- **Skinny-dipping!** Find a private (and safe!) location along a stream, ocean, or lake, take your clothes off, and get in. Closing your eyes, feel the water moving over your bare skin and imagine yourself becoming one with the water. Stay there until you feel no separation between yourself and the water. If you do not have access to a natural source of water, you can do this exercise in your bath.

Listen to your body; if the water is too cold or is unsafe, just meditate on the water's edge, allowing the voice of the water (babbling, crashing, or flowing) to connect you with its sacredness.

- **Water art:** Connect with your personal relationship to water by creating art inspired by water. Paint a picture of the ocean or a flowing stream, write a poem about your favorite lake, sculpt a rendition of waves out of clay, write a piece of music that imbues the spirit of water. Create, using water as your muse.

Water Birthing

Water birth is not a new-fangled hippie birthing movement — women have been giving birth in water (or at least immersing themselves in water for a portion of their birth) for thousands of years. It's believed that many pharaohs may have been born in water. Birthing in water lifts pressure off the laboring abdomen, opens the path for more efficient circulation of blood and oxygen, can diminish pain, softens the cervix and perineum, and helps to conserve and restore Mama's energy. If you're into the idea of using water as a member of your birth tribe, here are some suggestions to try out as you foster that relationship.

Be the Baby

"Being the baby" while you birth the baby will put you in the same state of fluid surrender your baby is in. During birth, babies don't do anything but accept the oxygen you send them and ride the fluid motions of your body that help them emerge. They absorbed this easy-going nature by floating in a warm pool of mama juice for nine-ish months. Recreating this environment for yourself during labor will deepen your connection and communication with your baby, will help you get out of the way of your surges by giving them oxygen instead of resistance, and will give your birthing muscles a much-appreciated reprieve.

Let the Water Lead You

Water moves where it needs to move. Allow this knowing to flow into you when you're in the water, prompting you to organically shift into the position your body needs to be in during each surge.

I attended the birth of a woman who swayed her hips between surges to release the buildup of tight energy that would collect in her hips during surges. Whenever a surge would roll through her, this swaying would immediately cease and she would contort into a rigid position and not move until the surge ended — she was also holding her breath. Her midwife drew a warm Epsom salt bath for her, we eased her into it between surges, and I encouraged her to continue the swaying during surges. The transformation was instantaneous. She began swirling her hips in the water through each surge, reporting that the gentle current her body created helped her stay in a pain-relieving rhythm. And she remembered how to breathe! Because she was now successfully moving the energy of the surge through her body while the surge was happening, she could rest in the water between surges rather than having to work out the tension.

Infuse It with Loving Pain Relief

Pretend that your warm bath is a huge vat of liquid narcotics. As you slip into it, the narcotics seep into your body and settle you into a warm and fuzzy, cotton-candy-like haze. In this yummy haze your mind floats off into a lovely dream state, while your body keeps on keepin' on. These pain-relieving effects are not just a trick of the mind; the warm water triggers a release of your natural pain relievers (endorphins) and blocks pain fibers from firing up. Warm baths can be so effective for pain relief that some refer to them as an *aquadural*.

Get Your Companion Involved

Many birth companions end up sitting nervously on the sidelines during birth, wishing they could do *anything* to assuage their lover's discomfort. They want to participate but often do not know what to do. Get your partner in the water. Have them throw on a Speedo, or better yet, skinny-dip (if you're both comfortable with that option), and sit with you in the tub, rubbing your lower back, cradling your head on their chest, kissing you or caressing your scalp through and between surges. The soothing effects of the water will be absorbed by your companion, serving to shift their energy to a frequency that will better support you.

If you desire a water birth and your care provider agrees this is a safe option for you, the energy you put into the rituals offered in this chapter will enrich your water birthing experience. Water will hold a new and reverent meaning for you, enhancing its powers to comfort you and support Baby's transition into new life.

What You'll Need

- The tub at the birthing center, hospital, or your home. You can also rent an inflatable birthing tub (and additional accessories) online. This option can be nice, as many birth-specific tubs have built-in seats and headrests for Mom.
- A close source of water so your supporters can add warm or cool water as desired.
- A thermometer to ensure water stays between 95 and 100 degrees Fahrenheit.
- Your water bottle. Sitting in warm water can dehydrate you, so take a few sips of water in between each surge.
- Washcloths to soak in cool water and place on your forehead to regulate your temperature. If desired, place three to five drops of lavender essential oil on the washcloth to enhance relaxation.
- Talk to your care provider about the option of using Epsom salt in the bathwater.

From Her Heart to Yours

I found labor to be intolerable until I sank into warm water. My midwife set the mood with an essential oil diffuser, twinkle lights (always a good idea), and meditation music, and she had my partner sink his nervous butt into the water with me. I had totally freaked him out by that point with my profane hollering and shallow breathing — he needed the bath *almost* as much as I did. Before entering the water, I felt so alone in my experience. No one could soothe me, and when people said, "You're doing this for your baby" I didn't feel any maternal revival of courage or determination — I just wanted it to stop.

The position I settled into in the water was on "all fours" with my head resting on my hub's shoulder, his hands cradling my belly. He would whisper encouragement in my ear through each surge, while rubbing my belly. That was when our trinity of love was born; we didn't have to wait for the actual moment of birth. I thank the water for removing my barriers to the bonding that opened me in a literal and figurative sense to my baby's birth.

— *S. R., Camarillo, California*

RIDDLE: I'm the liquid baby floats in, in the womb. What is my name?

Go to **YourSereneLife.wordpress.com/chapter-ten** and use the two-word riddle answer as your offer code to download the relaxation recording for this chapter!

CALL TO PLEASURE

- Buy a forty-ounce metal (or glass) water bottle.
- Drink at least one hundred ounces of water daily.
- Have the first twenty ounces within thirty minutes of waking.
- Tape the word *love* (or any other positive term) to the bottom of your bottle.
- Say a silent affirmation of gratitude with every sip.
- Set an hourly timer to remind you to drink water.
- Forge a stronger connection to the sacred nature of water by sending it appreciation as you bathe in it, creating water-inspired art, placing a "blessing-infused" natural object in a body of water, or performing any other ritual you feel deepens your respect for water.
- Discuss the option of water birth with your care provider, if you're into that idea.

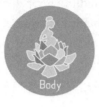

CHAPTER ELEVEN

WHAT IF I HAVE SPECIAL CIRCUMSTANCES?
Finding Calm in Chaos

JUST BREATHE: *Set the intention that your breath will deepen (rather than stop) when you're scared. Practice your "from chaos to calm" breathing — inhaling peace, calm, and love to a slow count of eight and releasing fear, tension, and stress to a slow count of eight. This is the breath you'll instantly shift into when you're faced with a scary thought or situation.*

Special circumstances, commonly referred to as *complications*, are the crux of our pregnancy fears. Women are afraid their body will decide to go this way instead of that, leading to a change in their plans. This chapter has landed in your hands to awaken faith in your body, mind, and spirit's ability to meet any change you may experience with courage and peace. We'll move through simple explanations of common pregnancy-related special circumstances, the frequently practiced solutions, and how you can maintain your inner state of calm throughout. My mission here is to remind you that you're not a patient, at the mercy of outside circumstances and medical care providers, but an empowered and knowledgeable woman capable of guiding your experience with your voice, heart, and innate sense of well-being.

I'm not going to get into the nitty-gritty of each special circumstance.

Your care provider will give you the most accurate information in regard to testing, symptoms, and treatments for any special circumstances you may experience. This space is going to focus on what you can do mentally and spiritually, alongside any medical treatments you may elect, to move through a special circumstance should one arise.

Complications vs. Special Circumstances

Complication: A circumstance that complicates something. A confused condition or state: "to add heightened complication." Synonyms: difficulty, problem, obstacle, hurdle, stumbling block, drawback, snag, catch, hitch, fly in the ointment (informal), headache.

Circumstance: A fact or condition connected with or relevant to an event or action. An event or fact that can cause, or help to cause, something to happen.

Which term sounds more serious, more menacing, more clinical? Which term do you think would bring more ease and well-being into your life?

The language we use has a direct effect on both our physiology and our psychology. Labeling unforeseen situations that could potentially occur in the course of your pregnancy, or birthing experience, as *complications* will add an unneeded level of difficulty and stress to your situation. Stuff happens, and because you likely have wonderful resources available to you, it is unlikely that any special circumstance that may arise will be too complicated. Even the "big" special circumstances can be moved through one small step at a time.

Unplanned Pregnancy

Holy sperm and egg, you're pregnant! If this juicy development wasn't on your five-year plan you may be freaking out. "Having kids" was so far down my list it was under "Win an Oscar" (ha!). I lost my mind, and my lunch, when I found out I was pregnant — but strangely, I also felt really happy. It may have taken a while for you to find that happy spot — heck, you still may be poking around for it — and that is *so* okay.

Shift Your Mentality to Adventure

Instead of focusing on the negative aspects of your unplanned pregnancy, think on how those barriers can be opportunities for birthing confidence, courage, connection, pride, and acceptance. So how about it? Think about the opportunities you could mine from this special life circumstance and write down your ideas. They don't even need to make sense — this is just intended to begin the process of loosening up your barriers so a bit of light can shine through.

One Small Daily Step

Once you give yourself space and self-compassion to name, accept, and release many of the *big* emotions conceived with unplanned pregnancy, you can begin to peel back the layers of the journey. Instead of paralyzing yourself in overwhelm over all that needs to be done before birth, take time to pull everything that needs to be done out of your head and onto a list. Include *everything* you currently feel you need to accomplish before Baby is born (e.g., telling your loved ones, choosing a care provider, making a baby registry, and taking classes about everything — hospital or home, placenta saving or trashing, etc.). Additional items will be added throughout the nine months; they too will eventually get done.

Now, tackle *one* task each day. If you're feeling overzealous because you threw some extra kale in your smoothie, go ahead and cross off two, but only if you are enthused by the notion.

Learn to Love Yourself Anyway

Most forms of special circumstances are introduced by Shame. He saunters in and hands you the unexpected news on a cold platter, then smirks and walks away. Even if your special circumstance has nothing to do with anything you did or did not do, it's still human nature to feel that this is "your fault" and that you deserve to feel shame. I call bull. You are amazing, and the only way to triumphantly move through the circumstance is to fire Shame by filling and surrounding yourself with an impenetrable shield of self-love and courage.

To build your shield, move through the following "Love Yourself" process. I encourage you to do this whenever you're faced with an unexpected slap from life.

1. Close your eyes and envision yourself, your baby, and your partner being surrounded by light and love. The light starts at the tops of your heads and slowly flows down every inch of your bodies until you're fully enveloped in it.

2. Now, talk with your partner and your care provider, together deciding on the best plan of action. Don't let your intuition be steamrolled; make sure you feel intuitively *good* about the actions you are going to take. These talks and decision-making sessions suck the power out of the unknown, the primary source of fear.

3. Throughout it all, breathe into your emotions.

4. Be here, in this present moment. Get in touch with the sights, sounds, textures, smells, and tastes surrounding you *now*. Don't allow your mind to wander to the thorny land of "what-ifs" — stand firm in the space where you presently are, where everything is exactly as it should be, even if it doesn't make sense to you. Just keep breathing yourself back into the present.

Gestational Diabetes

Gestational diabetes, also called "high blood sugar levels," occurs when the body cannot produce enough insulin, the hormone that aids the conversion of glucose (a type of sugar) to energy. This condition, when untreated, can cause your baby to grow too large and increase your risk of pre-eclampsia. Gestational diabetes happens, even to healthy chicks, and it does not mean you were diabetic before pregnancy or will be diabetic after giving birth.

How will you know if you have gestational diabetes? You'll be tested about twenty-four to twenty-eight weeks into your pregnancy; you'll be required to drink a syrupy drink, sit in a waiting room for an hour, and then have your blood drawn. Your care provider will give you the results at your next prenatal appointment. Your urine is also tested for sugar at each prenatal appointment.

Prevention

While gestational diabetes can happen to anyone, you can minimize your chances of developing it by maintaining a healthy meal plan, drinking plenty of water, exercising regularly, and taking steps to reduce your stress through self-hypnosis, meditation, and the "Love Yourself" process described in the previous section.

Group B Strep

This is *not* a sexually transmitted disease; I repeat, *not* an STD. Group B strep is a bacterium in the vagina, or the lower intestines, that has the potential to cause infection in Baby if she is exposed to it during birth. You will be tested for Group B strep around the thirty-sixth week of your pregnancy. Because this infection is "transient," meaning it comes and goes from the body, testing before the last leg of your pregnancy is often inaccurate.

About 40 percent of women have this bacterium present in their body and may choose to receive antibiotics during delivery, which will essentially make the Group B strep a nonissue. If you have Group B strep and you choose to receive antibiotics, you will receive a dose when your labor begins and every four hours thereafter, via IV, until your baby is born.

There are plenty of women who elect not to receive antibiotics — it's a personal choice and one I encourage you to work through with your care provider, making the decision that feels best to you.

Prevention

Give your vagina and digestive tract some tender care. Create a mix of two tablespoons of vinegar in one pint of water and pour a bit of it over your vulva every day for one week — doing this periodically throughout your pregnancy. (Do not put this mixture inside the vagina.) It's also crucial to build up good bacteria in your body. Give yourself food and drink rich in probiotics (like unsweetened Greek yogurt, kefir, sauerkraut, kimchee, and kombucha), and take probiotic supplements approved by your care provider. Boost these good bacteria carriers with echinacea tea, garlic, and foods rich in vitamins C and E. In addition, reduce your sugar intake; bad bacteria is in a love affair with processed sugar.

Premature Birth

For various reasons, some women have a higher likelihood of delivering their baby before Baby is considered "full term," that is, before thirty-seven weeks' gestation. Premature birth may occur from a special circumstance requiring that Mom be induced or receive a C-section, or it can occur from Baby naturally deciding to come early, for reasons your care provider can explain in better detail.

If you are having a happy and healthy birth, with a healthy baby, and your pregnancy is free of special circumstances, it's unlikely Baby is going to be born prematurely.

Navigating the Emotions of Having Baby Preterm

If your baby comes preterm, be gentle with yourself — you did all you could to have the healthiest possible pregnancy, and there is likely a reason (even if you can't see it) that your baby needed to arrive early. Torturing yourself about what you think you did wrong, or could have done better, is not going to give your new baby the love and nourishment he needs from you. Treat yourself as gently as you would your baby.

Having a baby prematurely can create a panicked feeling in you and your partner. You may feel you did not have time to prepare, and you may be faced with the challenges of more medical treatment and monitoring for your baby than would be required for a full-term baby. Practice open communication with your baby's care providers so you're able to feel connected to the experience and have optimal bonding with your little one.

Don't forget that you are allowed to feel; take the time you need to release your emotions by yourself, with your partner, or through a support group. Once you have released these emotions you will have more space to fill with love and acceptance for what is, and of course, for your baby.

Prevention

Follow these preventative measures, but equally important is practicing your ability to settle into The Now and give yourself unconditional love, so you can flow with any unforeseen events.

- See your care provider as soon as you suspect you're pregnant, or as soon as you begin trying to become pregnant. Continue this care on a regular basis.
- Take a daily prenatal vitamin before conception and throughout pregnancy.
- Ask your care provider if your medical history puts you at higher risk for preterm labor (i.e., prior early delivery, high blood pressure, carrying multiples, advanced maternal age, etc.). If you are at risk, your care provider can give you specific ways to minimize the risk.
- If you are at risk, visit the NICU at your local hospital and read about preterm infant care to minimize your fears of the unknown and bolster your sense of preparedness.
- Keep up on your probiotic-rich food and drink to minimize your chance of harmful bacteria being mischievous in your body.
- Because gum disease can trigger preterm labor, see your dentist regularly before and during pregnancy.
- Stay within a healthy range of weight (if you start your pregnancy at a healthy weight, you should gain twenty-five to thirty-five pounds). Eating small, regular, and healthy meals, exercising, and drinking your one hundred daily ounces of water will help regulate your weight.
- Know the signs of preterm labor — contractions that occur every ten minutes or more, pelvic pressure, cramping in the lower back or abdomen, and fluid leaking from the vagina. If you experience these symptoms, contact your care provider immediately, so they can hopefully stall labor.

Settle into Acceptance for What Is

Great peace comes when we learn to surrender to unforeseen circumstances that are out of our control. Life happens, often in ways that laugh at our preconceived plans. When fear of the unforeseen is replaced with curiosity for the unforeseen, which takes a lioness's share of courage, you're able not only to take preemptive action (i.e., by eating well, exercising, drinking water, getting plenty of rest) to avoid certain unsavory circumstances but also to hold a knowing that if life hits the fan, you have the gumption to navigate the shift, even if you hate it while it's happening. It's possible to "not be okay" with a negative circumstance while also growing, learning, and flowing with it.

Pre-eclampsia

Pre-eclampsia is usually composed of hypertension (high blood pressure), excessive swelling, and protein in the urine. Pre-eclampsia, like most special circumstances, can range from mild to severe. Because the symptoms of pre-eclampsia can be hard to detect, it is important to receive thorough prenatal care so your blood pressure and the protein levels in your urine can be monitored.

SIDE NOTE: *Because "protein in the urine" is a sign of pre-eclampsia, some women take this to mean they should restrict their protein intake during pregnancy. Don't do that. It is important to maintain a healthy diet, which includes healthy proteins (found in food like lean meats, eggs, nuts, dairy, and beans) to help prevent or reduce the severity of pre-eclampsia.*

Because high blood pressure can be caused by a constriction of the blood vessels, try this helpful self-hypnosis exercise: with your eyes closed, breathe deeply while envisioning your blood vessels being open and your blood freely and easily moving through them, spreading an ample supply of oxygen and nutrients throughout your body and your baby's. If you do experience pre-eclampsia, I urge you to use self-hypnosis in conjunction with whatever treatment you and your care provider select. (See chapter 12 for more on self-hypnosis.)

Breech Baby

Babies like to turn everything on its head, including themselves. Although most babies turn head down (vertex position) between weeks twenty-eight and thirty-two of gestation, some make the flip earlier, some later, and some flip back and forth. Your baby's head is the heaviest part of her little body, so gravity encourages her to flip if there is enough room for the flip to occur. One of the best ways to give your babe the room she needs is to reduce your stress. When you're stressed, your muscles contract, creating limited space in the uterus.

To stay relaxed, practice self-hypnosis structured around the following message: "My uterus expands, and Baby easily and effortlessly turns into the perfect position for birth. She is comfortable and safe in this position, and will remain here until it is time for her descent." Or something like that; use words that resonate with you.

What to Do When Baby Stays Head Up

If, at around thirty-seven weeks' gestation, your baby has ceased to turn, and if you've actively been practicing hypnosis methods to turn him, your care provider may recommend something called an external cephalic version (ECV) procedure. In this procedure, a care provider manually turns your baby by applying external pressure on your abdomen. ECV is not always successful, it is not risk free, and it does not guarantee your baby will stay in the head-down position if the procedure is successful. If you choose the ECV I recommend doing it in conjunction with hypnosis. A powerful combination can be listening to a "breech turn" hypnosis recording (a link can be found in the Resources section of this book) while the ECV procedure is being done. Not all women are candidates for ECV, and some feel it is too invasive; think through your options and follow your intuition.

A few less-invasive turn techniques are (1) getting on all fours and swirling your hips, (2) acupuncture, (3) walking, (4) swimming, and (5) trusting that your baby will turn when ready.

Need for Medical Pain Relief

No two people experience pain in exactly the same way, so let's squash the judgment toward women who elect artificial pain relief methods like an epidural because they feel they need it in their unique situation, as well as women who opt to go without painkillers because they feel that natural soothing techniques are enough for them.

Don't allow someone to shame you into not accepting (or accepting) painkillers because that's what *they* feel is the best option for you. Even if they've had ten babies, *you* are still the only one who knows how you're processing the sensations of labor.

Regardless of what type of birth you plan to have, I recommend discussing pain relief options with your care provider. Discussing the administration techniques, effects, and potential risks of all your options will allow you to go into childbirth with a stockpile of knowledge, should your plans shift when you're in the thick of labor. There are also certain medical conditions that would make you ineligible for various pain relief methods. Having these discussions *before* you're surging through contractions is much less stressful.

Need for Medical Induction

Here are three (of the many) nonmedical reasons I've heard from women requesting elective induction:

> "I want him born before May 21. There are enough Geminis in my family. They talk *so much.* I seriously can't handle another one."
> "My due date is on a full moon. I don't want to compete for attention if the birth center gets too full that night."
> "My mom is getting her boobs lifted next Tuesday, so I want to go into labor at least seventy-two hours before then, so she can be there."

I offer these examples to illustrate the difference between a "want" and a "need." While our wants are valid (even if other people struggle to see their validity), they don't trump "needs" when it comes to the birth of a baby. And really, the only need that qualifies in regard to the birth of a baby is a need for Mom and Baby to be healthy. So if there is no medical need for your baby to be born early, I implore you to hold off on medical induction — even if it's one of the hardest freakin' things you ever do. Why wait? Because *unnecessary* medical induction methods could lead you down paths you neither need nor want.

Make Sure It's Medically Necessary

If your care provider is the one urging you to medically induce, ask them questions until your mouth runs dry — who cares if they seem agitated? Don't accept medical induction until you feel it is the right choice for you. If there are medical concerns in play, have a thorough discussion with your care provider, ensuring that you end the convo with a complete understanding of the medical concerns, your options, and the risks and benefits of these options. If you and Baby are healthy, your body deserves the time it needs to go into labor when it's ready. And oh, my gosh — if your care provider wants to induce labor because they're leaving on an Alaskan cruise, find a new care provider!

Natural Induction Methods

When your baby is full term and your care provider gives you the go ahead, you can try the following options to encourage your baby and body to begin their trek into labor:

- **Spicy foods:** You know how spicy foods can sometimes get your bowels rollin'? Well, food with a kick can have the same effect on your uterus.
- **Sex — as much as you can handle:** Not only will this be one of the last times you can get your sex on without having a baby monitor by your head, but also your partner's semen contains prostaglandins (hormone-like compounds that help to ripen the cervix).
- **Boob massage, with an emphasis on the nipple:** This stimulation helps to release oxytocin, the same hormone that stimulates labor surges.
- **Red raspberry leaf tea:** This drink can help to galvanize the uterus into action.
- **Dates:** Begin eating about six dates a day four weeks before your Guess Due Time to encourage cervical dilation when the time is right.
- **Walking, dancing, swimming...get moving:** Physical movement can help Baby settle into the proper position for labor, potentially alerting the body that it's "go time."
- **Slough off stress:** You may want labor to begin *so badly* that you're actually impeding its ability to get going. When you're stressed, your body is tight and less likely to move into the flow of labor. Go get a prenatal massage, sniff some lavender oil, listen to a guided meditation, take a nap, write in a journal, do one of those nose strip things that pulls the blackheads out of your nose (Is this just relaxing for me?). Do anything that settles you back into the present moment.

- **Acupuncture, acupressure, or chiropractic work:** These techniques, when done by a professional, can help to align your body and energy with the journey of birth. Check with your care provider first!

Cesarean Birth

A cesarean birth can be just as spiritual and transformational as a vaginal birth. It's natural to feel some emotional deflation if you planned for a vaginal birth but because of medical circumstances end up with a cesarean birth. Know that you're allowed to feel bummed! But also know that you're allowed to feel psyched! Some women view this type of birth as a failure and believe they should be disappointed, even if their experience is pleasant. Entering the passage of birth with the knowledge that you will have the birth you are meant to have increases your chances of being satisfied (or even thrilled!) with your birth experience.

Some women require preplanned cesarean births because of certain medical conditions that make vaginal birth unsafe, or positional factors like baby being breech and the mother being uncomfortable with the prospect of having a vaginal breech birth. In other situations, mothers move into labor intent on having a vaginal birth, but end up needing a cesarean birth because of unforeseen medical circumstances that create a tenuous situation for Mother's or Baby's health. In either situation, it is good to have a basic knowledge of what you can expect from a cesarean birth, so your energies can be focused on staying calm and bonding with your baby during and after the procedure as opposed to worrying about what the heck that guy is doing with that scalpel. Visit the following link for a nonthreatening description of what to expect from a cesarean birth: YourSereneLife.wordpress.com/cesarean-birth.

How to Integrate with a Cesarean Birth

It can be difficult to reconcile your hopes with reality after an unplanned cesarean birth. You had visions of how your ideal birth would unfold and a different truth revealed itself. If you're struggling to come to terms with your birth, play around with exuding an attitude of gratitude even if you're initially faking it. Mentally (or verbally) repeat helpful and thankful affirmations, such as the following:

- I'm so grateful I had the medical care necessary to deliver a healthy baby.
- My baby had so many caring and skilled hearts and hands pour their energy into her entry into the world. We were both surrounded by so much love.
- Because I was free of the physical sensations of childbirth, my mind and spirit were able to play a bigger role in my baby's birth. Their focused attention surrounded Baby with love as she was lovingly lifted from my womb.

There is so much beauty and magic in the medical capabilities of the modern world — you can choose to relish the fact that these marvels were able to serve you in the highest sense, that of birthing life!

And, if you're still *so pissed* that you had to have a cesarean birth, feel that! Move through that regret, anger, or whatever else you're processing, *then* experiment with sentiments of gratitude.

You're Still Giving Birth!

Having surgery is intense — it puts your courage and your mind-body connection to the test, much like vaginal childbirth. You deserve to honor yourself. Don't allow anyone (including your inner voice, who can be an asshole) to tell you that you "didn't give birth" just because a surgeon was the one to physically help your baby emerge. You still spent forty-ish weeks growing the baby in your womb, and then you completely surrendered your body to the type of birth your baby needed to have. That is *epic*!

From Her Heart to Yours

I loved my cesarean birth. I had a room full of caring people who created an energy of excitement while prepping and performing my baby's birth. They made me feel special, not like a piece of meat on a table. They played the music I wanted, talked about what a sacred time this was for my family, and told me funny anecdotes about their own children. I know this is not the norm during cesarean

births, which is why I did everything I could to set up these conditions with my cesarean birth preferences. I had been planning for a
natural hospital birth, but when my baby had not turned by forty
weeks' gestation (and no doctors in my area would perform vaginal
breech births) the only option on my menu was a cesarean birth.
I had three days to pacify myself with this shift in birth plan and
do what I could to make it "my own." My requests on my cesarean
birth plan were honored, and I still feel so much love for everyone
who was in that room.

— *K. M., Santa Barbara, California*

RIDDLE: What type of massage can naturally induce labor? Hint:
The word starts with a *B*.

Go to **YourSereneLife.wordpress.com/chapter-eleven** and use the
one-word riddle answer as your offer code to download the relaxation recording for this chapter!

CALL TO PLEASURE

❧❧❧

If a special circumstance enters your reality, follow these "Love Yourself"
steps to navigate the shifts in your experience with a core sense of peace and
empowerment.

- Cry. Rage. Bang on the proverbial wall. Let out any and all of the
  "yuck stuff" that wants to express itself. The negativity doesn't fester
  into something harmful if it's able to have a voice — and its voice
  often becomes softer after it lets out the initial wail.

- After you feel clear of a majority of the initial gloom, envision surrounding your baby, your partner, and yourself in light and love.
  Then...

- Talk with your partner and care provider, together deciding on the best plan of action. Don't let your intuition be steamrolled; make sure you feel intuitively *good* about the actions you are going to take.
- Breathe.
- Be here, in this present moment. Get in touch with the sights, sounds, textures, smells, and tastes surrounding you *now*. This allows you to cease living in the "what if."

CHAPTER TWELVE

HYPNOSIS:
Traveling Within

JUST BREATHE! *Each time you cycle through a breath, allow your inhalation and exhalation to stretch into time, taking you deeper and deeper. As your breathing goes deeper and longer, notice your eyelids becoming heavier and heavier, eventually closing. Take a moment to rest here before moving into this chapter.*

Hypnosis is a focused state of relaxation that can awaken your best Self; it has the power to replace negative behaviors, beliefs, and thought processes with positive alternatives. This chapter conveys the principles of hypnosis, explains how to achieve self-hypnosis, and articulates the balancing and harmonizing power this intentional mental reprogramming practice delivers. So, whether you are well versed in hypnosis, a skeptic, or somewhere in between, read on to learn about the state we all enter, every day.

What Is Hypnosis?

When guided into hypnosis by a professional hypnotherapist, you enter an intentional state of calm that reprograms your subconscious mind by canceling negative beliefs and behaviors and replacing them with positive ones. Your critical mind, the filter between your conscious and subconscious mind, usually rejects these positive suggestions because of deeply rooted be-liefs. During guided hypnosis you are in a heightened state of suggestibility, which allows the positive suggestions to bypass the critical mind, enter your subconscious mind, and take lasting effect.

You may be surprised to hear that you're in the state of hypnosis every day. You know that fuzzy la-la land you're in between waking up and falling asleep? When you're not fully awake, but not fully asleep? That's hypnosis. You know that feeling you get when you're driving home and you check out from the experience of driving because your mind starts dissecting the passive-aggressive convo you had with your boss? And you safely pull into your driveway but don't remember the last ten minutes of your drive? That's hypnosis. You know that blissed-out, timeless vibe you flow into when you're in "the zone"? That's hypnosis.

These everyday "dreamy" states are all hypnosis. There's nothing supernat-ural about it; it's an organic space for the mind-body-spirit to inhabit — the three of them enjoy playing together there. The juicy opportunities living in hypnosis start to flow when the state of hypnosis is intentionally (as opposed to unconsciously) entered, and you or a trained hypnotherapist have specific positive messages and images to plant in the subconscious mind.

I'm a Certified Hypnotherapist, and I often work with pregnant women to overcome their fears surrounding pregnancy, birth, and motherhood. Here's how it works: We deal primarily in the positive, rarely putting em-phasis on the negative. This is not the type of inner work that requires you to relive that time you were humiliated in front of your third-grade class because you forgot how to spell your name during the spelling bee. (I *knew* how to spell my name; the pressure just got to me.) Before, and sometimes during, hypnosis we briefly name the negative beliefs, behaviors, attitudes, or thought processes we want to change, then shift focus to the positive alter-natives we prefer. We take those specific positive alternatives, enter the comfy state of hypnosis, and reprogram the subconscious mind.

When this state is purposefully entered, the potential holistic effects you can create are limitless — you can cancel mental blocks, nurture your soul, heal your body, and transform your life — all fun stuff that also makes babies really chill and happy. And to support the relaxation recordings (a form of hypnosis) you've already been listening to, I'm going to teach you how to intentionally put yourself into hypnosis.

Misconceptions

If you still have a weird taste in your mind because you're envisioning college students quacking on a stage as a hypnotist barks commands at them, let me give you a mental breath mint. Hypnosis is not mind control, it does not put you in a state where you feel out of control, and it rarely causes amnesia. (And stage hypnotists know how to select members of a crowd who are highly suggestible and up for some *voluntary* quacking.)

If you choose to move beyond the self-hypnosis techniques you'll learn in this chapter and seek out the services of a hypnotherapist, be assured that your subconscious mind is going to accept only those suggestions offered by the hypnotherapist that you feel comfortable with. If they were to ask you about your most embarrassing moment or your bank account number (they won't) while you're under hypnosis, you would have the choice to stand up, flip them the bird, and walk out. You have full use of your facilities during all forms of hypnosis.

Theory of Mind

So what's up with your mind? What's it composed of? What's the deal with that iceberg image commonly used to portray the structure of the mind? How does hypnosis affect the iceberg?

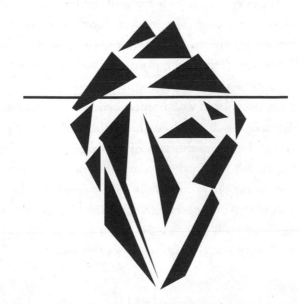

There are three primary areas of the mind that need to be affected for an individual to enter the state of hypnosis. In addition there is a fourth area that is occasionally tickled by hypnosis. About 12 percent of the mind makes up your conscious mind, and 88 percent is your subconscious mind.

1. **The conscious mind — the exposed tip of the iceberg:** This is the holding area for the memories you have gathered in the last hour and a half; certain memories from before that time start to trickle down into the deeper vaults of the mind. The conscious mind is also where your willpower, reason, logic, and decision making live.

2. **The critical area — the veil of water separating the visible tip of the iceberg from the hidden hunk of ice below:** The critical area of the mind lives in both the conscious and the subconscious areas of the mind. It retains memories for twenty-four hours before they are either rejected or dropped down into the subconscious mind for long-term storage. The critical area acts as a filter between the conscious and subconscious mind. The critical mind is what we want to make porous during hypnosis so positive suggestions can drop into the subconscious mind without too much dilution.

3. **Modern memory — a big ole hunk of the hidden ice, also called** *the subconscious mind*: The modern memory is the area of the subconscious mind that holds memories from conception to the present moment. This is the main area we want to access during hypnosis because this is where negative, deep-seated beliefs and behaviors can be replaced with positive beliefs and behaviors.

4. **Primitive area — the bottom tip of the underwater portion of the iceberg:** The primitive area of the mind is the other part of the subconscious mind, where your fight, flight, or freeze reactions (common during birth) come from. The primitive area of the mind will react only when triggered (usually through regression), while in the state of hypnosis (which is uncommon), or when it is seriously threatened — or *thinks* it is being seriously threatened.

What Does It Feel Like?

"Will I go into a coma?"

"Will I float out of my chair?"

"Will my eyes roll back so far in my head they'll get stuck like that?"

All questions I've been asked by clients (mostly clients under the age of twelve). But my adult clients also come in wary of what to physically expect from hypnosis. As I previously mentioned, hypnosis is a state you enter every day, which means it will be a familiar state for your body.

In the lighter stages of hypnosis, you will typically experience rapid eye movement, followed by a deepening of the breath, then deep relaxation where you will be highly receptive to verbal suggestions. You will not be in a "trance," you'll just be really relaxed. It's like receiving an emotional and spiritual massage that your body also reaps rewards from, even though it is never touched during hypnosis (with the occasional exception of the hypnotherapist touching the center of the client's forehead, or placing slight pressure on their shoulder). You will remain in complete control of your mental and physical facilities during hypnosis, you'll just be more okay with everything loosening up a bit.

Self-Hypnosis vs. Hetero-Hypnosis

Self-hypnosis and hetero-hypnosis both achieve similar results; they're just delivered in different formats. During hetero-hypnosis, where someone else guides you into hypnosis, the hypnotherapist has a clearly organized intention for what and how they are going to deliver various positive suggestions to your subconscious mind, and they utilize their ability to disorganize your conscious mind to take you to a suggestible hypnotic state. During self-hypnosis, you begin with an organized conscious mind and intentionally take yourself into the state of hypnosis while consciously delivering your positive suggestions. In self-hypnosis, you are both the hypnotherapist and the client.

The relaxation recordings that go along with this book are examples of hetero-hypnosis. I recommend you listen to these as often as you can while sitting in a quiet and comfortable location. And please, for the love of aching, pregnant bladders everywhere, get up and pee as many times as you need during the recording.

Swapping the Negatives with the Positives

Hypnosis can work for you or against you. During times in your life when you unintentionally slipped into a state of hypnosis, you were likely more susceptible to any messages, both negative and positive, offered to you — whether those came from others or, most commonly, from your inner critic. When the messages absorbed were negative, they likely wiggled down into your subconscious mind, eventually sprouting beliefs, attitudes, and actions that do not serve you. That's why it's not enough to just enter hypnosis and receive some positive messages that sound good — it's important to first name what *isn't* working. What beliefs are you sick of gnawing on? What actions do you recognize as harmful, but can't figure out how to quit? What attitudes about pregnancy and childbirth are blocking you from enjoying the journey?

You can spend hours psychoanalyzing the limiting seeds living in your subconscious mind, *or* you can decide what their positive opposites are and allow them to swap places, through self-hypnosis. For example, I often eat ice cream as a way to "check out" from my stressors, but when I do that I feel lethargic and regretful afterward. The positive opposite of this could be going for a walk when I need to check out. So, during self-hypnosis I could give myself the suggestion, "When I'm feeling overwhelmed and want to check out, I go for a walk — and it works." There's no need to make myself hate ice cream, or to feel shame for using it as an emotional aid. I just give myself something else to do, something positive, whenever the emotions that commonly push me to eat ice cream pop up. There's no need to pour poison on the "bad" to make space for the good.

Here are two more pregnancy-specific suggestions:

1. **Limiting message:** "Every time I think about childbirth, I envision traumatic scenes of women screaming and twisting in pain. This makes me cringe at the thought of giving birth."
    Positive swap: "I release my old beliefs about childbirth; I don't want them anymore, I don't need them anymore. Now, when I think about childbirth, I envision myself and my birth companion,

peacefully moving through all phases of childbirth, breathing easy, making informed decisions, exuding courage, and even smiling and laughing a bit! These visions are manifesting my ideal birth."

2. **Limiting message:** "My body is not strong enough to grow and birth a baby. I've had health issues in the past and feel inadequate in my body's abilities."

    Positive swap: "My body grows stronger every day as I feed it nourishing food, water it with fresh liquid, and move it in loving ways. The struggles my body had in the past made it more wise and capable because it now knows what *not* to do. My body fully supports me and my baby in pregnancy, birth, and beyond."

There is a lovely flip side to every challenge living in your subconscious mind. Name the "yuck," sprinkle it with some mental "yum" while in hypnosis, and joyfully observe the beauty that grows as a result.

How to Practice Self-Hypnosis

When you don't have a relaxation recording or a hypnotherapist on hand, it's important to learn how to take yourself "there" on your own.

1. First, I want you to select a "physical sensation" word that you enjoy feeling. Maybe a physical sensation you experience when you hear great news, or complete a satisfying workout. For example, I always feel a pleasing lightness after I leave a yoga class.

    Examples:

    *   *Grounded*
    *   *Tingling*
    *   *Vibrating*
    *   *Weightless*
    *   *Buzzing*

2. Next, select an "emotional" word describing what you feel you need more of.

    Examples:

    *   *Confidence*
    *   *Happiness*

- *Calmness*
- *Strength*
- *Power*

3. Now, decide what limiting belief, attitude, or action you want to swap out during this session (just do one at a time). Using the limiting birthing messages examples previously discussed, you could set the intention that during this self-hypnosis you are going to replace the traumatic birth images swimming in your subconscious mind with peaceful images (of you!) moving through a beautiful birthing experience.

4. Then, close your eyes (after you've read this!) and focus on your breath. Inhale to a steady count of eight and exhale to an equally slow count of eight.

5. Take a few moments to concentrate on your breath and envision relaxation flowing into you with each inhalation, and all stress streaming out of you with each exhalation.

6. Place your attention on any area of your being that is holding tension and send a loving breath to it, releasing the tension.

7. Now, place your focus on the "physical sensation" word you selected. If your word was *tingling*, begin to notice a tingling sensation washing through your body. Stay with this tingling sensation, and let it continue through your self-hypnosis session.

8. When you're ready, envision yourself standing at the top of a flight of twenty stairs. Imagine walking down each step, while counting from twenty to zero in your head. You will fall deeper and deeper into a relaxed state of hypnosis. When you reach the bottom step at the count of zero, you will be in the deepest state of relaxation you've ever known. You're tingling even more.

9. Now, imagine the "emotional" word you selected and feel it coursing through you, and radiating from you. If your word was *confidence*, feel that confidence, let it soak into your mind, body, and spirit, let it replace any negative seeds living in your subconscious mind with confidence. You are the source of pure confidence. Be with this confidence. If you have trouble connecting with a sense of

confidence, remember an event in your life when your confidence was high and relive it in your mind.

10. As you're tingling with confidence in this safe space in your subconscious mind, bring up the limiting message (image, belief, etc.) that you want to replace, and begin the replacement by letting images or feelings (or both) of the positive replacement flow through you. Experience everything attached to the positive replacement as long as you like. For example, if you want to replace the limiting message that your baby will not fit through your pelvis on the day of birth, imagine the opposite of that scene: an image of your baby easily traveling down and out of your pelvis. Notice the feelings of relief and joy attached to the positive scene.

11. When you feel ready to resume your natural state of alertness, slowly count yourself up from zero to five, visualizing yourself walking up five stairs that lead back to your conscious mind. As you count up, you will feel a rejuvenating light entering your being, you will become aware of your surroundings, and you will feel whole, confident, and wide awake. (If you are using self-hypnosis to fall asleep, skip this part.)

From Her Heart to Yours

I had a partial hysterectomy when I was twenty-two and thought I was destined to cry in longing every time I saw a baby. As the IVF industry evolved I saw my destiny brighten. When I was thirty-two, my husband and I went through the nerve/gut/heart-wrenching experience of discovering whether I had any viable eggs — I did! We yelled a "Screw it!" to the universe and jumped into the process of baby-making (with the help of a bunch of people who wear white coats). My eggs were scrambled up with my hubby's sperm to make embryos, and these embryos were implanted in the healthy uterus of a gestational surrogate. The embryo accepted the uterus and baby-growing magic commenced.

Then, I totally freaked out. I had been so focused on "action!"

throughout our IVF journey I hadn't had time to sit with my shifting reality — the pregnancy created the space for that sitting, and it was awful. My emotions were battered with thoughts of the baby not bonding with me because I wasn't growing her body in mine, mourning for the loss of my uterus, dread that my daughter's lovely surrogate would make a health misstep and trigger a cascade of complications, and other fun paranoid stuff. My husband recommended hypnotherapy and I called him a hippie — but I tried it. I loved it. I felt physically lighter each time I left my weekly session, and happily became addicted to the self-hypnosis techniques I was taught. Hypnosis didn't make me hack up my doubts with painful effort, it just gave me other options to take the place of the doubts. I'm now my baby's favorite person, and the feeling is mutual.

— *H. I., Ventura, California*

RIDDLE: What do you call a professional who is trained to relax people, help them drift into their subconscious mind, and guide them through the replacement of negative messages with positive alternatives?

Go to **YourSereneLife.wordpress.com/chapter-twelve** and use the one-word riddle answer as your offer code to download the relaxation recording for this chapter.

CALL TO PLEASURE

* Listen to a relaxation recording daily.
* If you're interested in exploring hetero-hypnosis further, find a local hypnotherapist you connect with.
* Practice self-hypnosis!

    1. Select your "physical sensation" and "emotional sensation" words and the negative belief you are going to swap with a positive belief.

2. Close your eyes and focus on your breath.

3. Focus on your "physical sensation" word. Let it flow through you and stay with you.

4. Envision yourself walking down twenty stairs into your subconscious mind.

5. When you reach the bottom, allow your "emotional sensation" word to fill you.

6. Swap the negative belief you are working with in this session with its positive opposite.

7. Remain here and drift into sleep, or count yourself up and out from zero to five.

CHAPTER THIRTEEN

PAST LIFE REGRESSION:
Opening the Eyes of Your Past

JUST BREATHE: *As you slowly inhale, envision new space being created in your mind, where openness for fresh ideas and perspectives can live. Allow this space to expand further with every inhalation.*

From My Heart to Yours: I Was Afraid to Raise a Boy Because I Wasn't Good at Being One

I lost "all of it" when I found out I was having a boy. I had been certain I was having a girl. I *knew* how to be a girl, so I felt confident in my ability to raise a girl. But no, there was a penis growing inside me. I had been building a bond with my "sex unknown" baby for the whole fifteen weeks since my pregnancy test, but this bond dissolved when I discovered the sex at my twenty-week ultrasound. I felt guilty, but could not shake my aversion to penis-growing.

I cried all this out to my hypnotherapist, who asked me plenty of questions about my current life in an attempt to help us figure out why I was having such a strong reaction to this "not a girl" news. We found nothing. I have a loving male partner and father, no history of any serious issues with other men — nada, I'm cool with dudes. So she suggested we try a past life regression (PLR). I was so down.

I subscribe to the idea of past lives, I lap it up — it makes sense to me and it feels good to me. So I went into the experience open, excited to relive some fabulous past life where I was a fairy queen. But there were no fairies.

My first vision was of big, hairy man-hands, then giant, gritty work boots. I immediately felt uncomfortable — I was not supposed to be a *man*. But there I was, a giant, lumbering, hairy guy. The life of this man was lonely and dark; he lost his parents as a baby and became a forgotten orphan. His adult life was just as bleak. He was a man soft in spirit who attracted animals, but few humans. He died alone in a dusty street from a sudden and smooth heart attack.

Then, my hypnotherapist brought me back.

I cried for twenty minutes after the session, and then, when the tears cleared, I started laughing. I felt so light. I no longer felt afraid to have a baby boy, and I was free of my initial guilt. I didn't pick apart the details of the PLR to determine what about it had a direct correlation to my current life; I just allowed the sensations to wash over me — sensations composed of relief, hope, understanding, connection, oneness, and acceptance.

Did you know you might have lived hundreds, maybe even thousands, of lives before this one? Ma-a-ay-be. Whether you fully subscribe to this belief, are tinkering around with the idea, or laughed when you read the first line of this paragraph, there are many therapeutic benefits to the exploration found in PLR therapy.

PLR is a hypnotherapy modality that guides your subconscious to a past time in which you may have lived. It has the potential to reconnect you with loved ones, heal current traumas, mend unexplainable wounds, release the fear of death, and elicit remarkable epiphanies.

In this chapter I'm going to provide the knowledge and tools you can use to safely explore your own potential past lives, when you're ready.

Follow Your Intuition — It's Okay to Wait

A past life regression could bring up uncomfortable emotions in you — what the process often reveals are the more intense moments of potential past lives because that's where the most profound messages live. While the deepest healing and discovery often come through processing emotional confusion or discomfort, that might not be where you feel comfortable going with baby in tow, and that's okay. If you have the desire to explore PLR but feel you might be blocked from the full experience while pregnant, you can wait until after childbirth to experience it.

But if you're feeling unexplained anxieties, fear, or other constrictive feelings that have not been able to be released by other methods, and you feel these barriers will hold you back from experiencing your best possible pregnancy and childbirth, it may serve you to explore PLR therapy now. Make a thorough plan with the PLR practitioner you select in regard to how deep you want to go, the method you feel comfortable using to be regressed to the past life, and special words or touches (such as a firm touch to the shoulder) that will be your signal to quickly and easily come out of the PLR should it become too emotionally intense for you.

Do what *you* feel is best for your specific needs, remaining open to exploration yet committed to not pushing yourself further than you're comfortable going. It's natural to want to take baby steps when you're growing a baby.

Choose the Right Practitioner

A pivotal factor in your PLR experience is your connection to and comfort with the practitioner. Select an individual you feel safe and open with, going to a few standard hypnotherapy sessions with them before deciding to enter the epic voyage of a PLR. Here are a few action steps to take, and factors to consider, before asking them to be the one to join you in opening up your soul's memory.

- Ask questions until the water in your mind runs clear.
- Tune in to how open you feel around this person. If you're hesitant to share certain things, it may be difficult for you to open up during the PLR.
- How do you feel about the physical environment of their office? Ask if that is the space where they will do the PLR. If not, ask to see that space. If you don't feel good in the space, it may not be the right place for you to past-life regress.
- Do they have a soft and maternal energy? Many of my pregnant

clients have mentioned that this type of energy makes them feel more comfortable in this vulnerable stage of their life.

- Before undertaking the PLR, make sure the practitioner fully explains the step-by-step process they will use to regress you, what you can expect from the experience, and how they will be supporting you through the journey. This pre-regression discussion usually takes a minimum of an hour. You can ask as many questions as you need during this time and fully express your goals for the regression (e.g., a need to release fears of childbirth, desire to reconnect with a loved one who has passed away, explanation and release of a phobia, etc.).
- Make sure you inform the hypnotherapist that you are pregnant, and ensure that they're comfortable working with you while you're in this heightened state of mental, physical, and spiritual awareness and vulnerability.
- Hire someone only if you feel excited about the prospect of them supporting you in a PLR.

To find a practitioner, I recommend asking trusted friends and family for recommendations — personal referrals rock. If you don't receive any recommendations, do an online search for PLR practitioners in your area and call many of them, until you settle on the few you would like to meet in person. I would avoid doing the PLR over the phone; this is a very intimate experience that should be done in person, and if you need to be brought out of hypnosis before the end of the session, it's important the practitioner share your physical space.

You Just Need to Bring Your Curiosity

If you're interested in exploring the process of a PLR but don't know if you fully believe in the concept of past lives, that's okay — you can still benefit from the experience as long as you bring your curiosity and openness. Some choose to experience a PLR for religious or spiritual reasons, or a deep need to explore their core Self. Whether or not they've totally bought into it, the one thing they have in common is curiosity and a need to learn more about their authentic selves.

During the PLR it's very common to question or doubt what you're experiencing. For example, your inner critics may pipe up with, "Is this real? Am I making up everything I'm seeing or sensing? Is this a total sham?" These are common quips from your inner gang of cynics, and there is nothing wrong with them. It's natural to question anything that is intangible.

You get to choose what you want to believe; maybe some of what you're experiencing is being totally fabricated by your mind, maybe some of it really is being pulled from a past life. And you know what? It doesn't matter if it's "real" or not, as long as you stay open to the experience, holding on to what deeply affects you, piques your interest, or makes you *feel* something — and release the rest. There is no right or wrong way to experience a PLR.

The Past Life Regression Process

Most PLR sessions take place after you've had a few traditional hypnotherapy sessions with your hypnotherapist of choice — ensuring the establishment of a comfortable rapport, a base for your knowledge in regard to hypnosis, and a customized hypnotic foundation on which you and your hypnotherapist can build.

Here's what you can expect before and during the PLR session:

1. The PLR practitioner will likely ask you to fill out a questionnaire and send it in ahead of time, or bring it with you to the session. This questionnaire will address topics such as names and details of important people in your life (past or present); what you hope to gain from the experience; locations, cultures, or languages you've always had an unexplained fascination with; and other things that will help guide the practitioner during the session. They will not lead you with this information, they'll just know to dig deeper with questions should one of these bits of information arise during the session.

2. The PLR session typically lasts three to four hours — significantly longer than the typical one-hour hypnotherapy session.

3. Your practitioner will then discuss the PLR process with you so you feel prepared and comfortable with how they will guide you through this journey.

4. The practitioner will then have you use the bathroom (few things are as distracting as a full bladder) and settle you into a reclining

chair, maybe placing a blanket on you if you're comfortable with that. They will then set the mood by lowering the lights.

5. They'll spend a minimum of thirty minutes taking you through a progressive relaxation, helping your mind, body, and spirit relax.

6. Next, they'll use the technique they previously explained to you to regress you back to a life in which you may have lived.

7. Once you're in the past life experience, they'll guide you by asking nonleading questions (questions that do not plant information in your mind, but create the space for you to explain your experience).

8. During the past life portion of the session, the practitioner will likely take notes and make a recording so you can explore everything you experienced at a later time.

9. At the end of each life you explore, your practitioner will safely lead you through the death experience. Depending on time, and how you're handling the journey, the practitioner may lead you into another past life, or slowly bring you back to your current surroundings.

10. After the PLR is complete, the two of you will reflect upon your experience, your questions, and your potential epiphanies. The reflection time will also give you the opportunity to reorient yourself with your current time and space.

Healing Your Birth Story

A common method of regressing to a past life is to scan back through your current life, moving through your birth experience and journey in the womb before entering a life that came before that. This exploration into your birth and gestation journey can be deeply healing, especially if you had a traumatic birth experience. It's believed that we remember our birth experience on a cellular level, so a journey full of trauma can translate into your current birth holding an energy of fear and doubt. Many times, all that's needed to clear that energy is to (safely) re-view your birth journey. I say "re-view" instead of "re-live" because any traumatic experiences you move through in a PLR can be witnessed from a safe distance, as if you were watching a movie or floating above the action as a curious observer. You don't need to re-live the trauma (which is why death transitions during a PLR often feel very liberating, rather than distressing).

If you're interested in regressing back to your birth but don't wish to go farther than that, there are many hypnotherapists who specialize in birth regressions; just use the criteria previously listed to find a practitioner you sync with.

Safety Measures

While a PLR is physically safe, you want to *feel* safe as well. Here are a few things to consider before beginning a PLR to establish a sense of safety, which is an integral requirement of staying open to the experience.

- The practitioner should not use anything but their voice and your mind to regress you. The one exception is the use of a blanket for warmth.
- Ensure the practitioner thoroughly covers their techniques for bringing you out of hypnosis should you begin to experience an adverse reaction.
- If you have allergies to any essential oils or candles (or you just don't like them!), tell the practitioner so they do not use any of these devices during your session.
- Verify that the practitioner has had adequate training in the field of hypnotherapy — specifically in PLRs.
- While there are many "DIY" PLR recordings and scripts online, I recommend moving through this process with a trained professional.
- Do not do a PLR if your health is in a tenuous state. It will be more difficult for you to concentrate on the regression.

RIDDLE: What is the name of the relaxation technique that takes a minimum of thirty minutes and that a hypnotherapist uses before beginning the process of regressing you into a past life?

Go to **YourSereneLife.wordpress.com/chapter-thirteen** and use the two-word riddle answer as your offer code to download the relaxation recording for this chapter!

CALL TO PLEASURE

Spend some time meditating on whether or not a past life regression, or birth regression, is something you're interested in. If the answer is no, that's okay! If the answer is yes, continue with the following recommendations:

1. Ask friends and family members to recommend hypnotherapists who are trained in PLR. Or do a search online for PLR practitioners.
2. Then, thoroughly interview a minimum of three practitioners, settling on the one you feel most comfortable with.
3. See the chosen practitioner for at least one standard hypnotherapy session before scheduling the PLR.
4. Enter the PLR with curiosity and a knowing that you do not need to move through it if you begin to feel uncomfortable. Follow your instincts.

THIRD TRIMESTER
COUNTDOWN
to
BIRTH

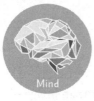

CHAPTER FOURTEEN

HOW TO ORGANIZE THE BEDROOM — WHERE THE NEW KIND OF MAGIC HAPPENS

Just Breathe. Take in a long inhale, imagining the essence of simplicity flowing into you — whatever that feels like for you. Allow each inhalation to deepen your commitment to simplifying your physical space, and each exhalation to release your emotional attachment to stuff and to your home's status quo.

Your bedroom should be a sanctuary of simplicity, offering an empty space for you to pour out the struggles of your day and recharge. When you enter this simple sanctuary, you will feel relief, safety, and a love for every color, image, and object you see. This is your cozy space to nuzzle into when life is being a demanding shrew.

Let's work together to get your space into the category of "sanctuary" by utilizing some of the feng shui tips previously mentioned — good air, lighting, clutter-clearing, and color — as well as employing optimal storage solutions, creating "energy nooks," leaving out stressful items, creating a "flow of energy" furniture arrangement, and learning how to maintain that essence of *simplicity*. That is the key word in this process — if you stay in the mind-set of simplicity you cannot fail. Live simply.

If your babe will have his own nursery, you can use many of these techniques to create a serene nursery. But, whether he'll have his own room or not, Baby will be spending time in your bedroom, so you might as well make it fun for all ages.

Start with a Dream

When you have surges of hormones, and thoughts of breast pump selection are overwhelming your system, it can be difficult to paint an image of what your ideal sanctuary of simplicity will look like. Let the internet paint it for you; search for inspiration in design magazines or online. The idea is not to duplicate the totally gorgeous but usually impractical bedroom the internet dangles in front of you, but to use it as a spark of inspiration for your unique bedroom vision. And throw the latest fads in color and style out the plantation-shuttered window — the only people the room needs to *feel good* to are you, your partner, and your sprout. Let this vision be your guide as you flow through the following sanctuary-making suggestions.

Feng Shui Reminders

- **Clutter-clearing:** Remember, keep your life simple and serenity will follow. The primary resource your baby (and your Self!) will need for a happy life is *you* — allow that idea to free you from a need for superfluous stuff. We have been led to believe that our lives will become richer with more stuff, when in reality life just becomes heavier. Go through your bedroom and donate or throw away any items that do not bring you immense joy or value. Touch each item. If you notice a sense of struggle or indecision come over you when you hold it, honor it for having served you, then let that sucker go. Clearing your bedroom of all unneeded, unused, and unloved items will cleanse your canvas, inviting in fresh loving energy.
- **Open-window policy:** Purchase and install window guards in all the windows in your bedroom that can open. When the weather is nice, open them up, taking a moment to close your eyes and feel the fresh air moving in and out of your nose. To inspire you to open the windows, purchase light and beautiful curtains that will float in the breeze that's pulled into your space. In the center of the curtains you can hang a light-refracting crystal that will transform

rays of light into dancing glimmers of creative and whimsical energy. (My son calls the rainbows birthed from the crystal in his window his "angels." And watching a kid chase rainbow angels on the ground is hilarious.)

- **Nourishing lighting:** Nothing kills the sanctuary vibe of a bedroom like crummy lighting. Turn off the overhead light whenever possible, instead opting for natural light during the day and three lamps, placed at two or three different levels, in the evening.

- **Soothing colors:** The most soothing colors for bedroom walls are skin tones ranging from light caramel to deep brown, but if you find those hues lean too far into the "snore-zone" (which is kind of the point, right?) select a soft tone of your favorite color. The same color rule applies to bedding and to any other prominent fixture in the room. To add pops of color, hang a few favorite photos or paintings in aesthetically pleasing frames around the room, being sure not to overdo it. Select images with colors that evoke the emotions you would like to fill your bedroom with — go to page 31 for a reminder about the energy awakened by different colors.

Storage

Continue the legacy of simplicity passed down by your clutter-clearing efforts and find a home for your bedroom essentials. I recommend displaying only a few key items that are meant to be seen and admired often. Everything else should be nestled away in an out-of-sight location. Here are a few storage options:

- **Nightstand:** Ideally, your nightstand has a pull-out drawer. If not, place an attractive bin here to hold your bedtime desirables (e.g., glasses, book, lotion, lip balm, lavender oil, lube?).

- **Under the bed:** The philosophy of feng shui recommends you store nothing under the bed, allowing energy to freely move below it. I understand this concept, but I also have a nest-like (i.e., miniscule) bedroom with minimal storage and need somewhere besides the shelves on my wall to store my underwear. If you also live in a tiny nest, place pull-out drawers specifically designed for under-bed storage below your sleep zone. Energy might get stuck down there, but at least it will have an organized space to chill in.

- **Furniture storage:** There are many bed frames, chairs, footstools, and other forms of furniture that double as storage. If you'll be purchasing new bedroom furniture, select options that allow you to hide stuff inside them.

- **Wall storage:** If possible, reserve wall storage for books, photos, and other items that can easily appear organized and are pleasant to look at. If you must store other items (I'm looking at you, underwear) on wall storage, place them in attractive canvas (or metal, or whatever) bins or baskets that fit on the shelving.

- **Bins and baskets:** I ordered twenty beige canvas bins from my favorite online mega-store when I was pregnant. I use them in my closet, bedroom, kitchen, living room, and garage; I even have one in my car. If in doubt, put your stuff in a pretty bin.

Energy Nooks

Each nook in your bedroom should exude a special blend of energy that facilitates the main activity experienced in that space. For example, creating a comfortable sleeping nook with plush textures and soft colors will promote a calming energy in that zone, putting you in the frame of mind to slip into …sex? Just kidding. *Sleep.* We just want sleep. Your creativity nook can be filled with inspirational energy by adding a cozy chair and a display of your favorite books, journals, and stimulating images that galvanize you into exploration and creation.

Here are the primary zones to consider designing in your nest:

- **Sleeping:** The quickest way to kill the peaceful energy in your sleep nook is to bring a pile of bills into it. Reserve your bed for bonding, sleeping, and sex. Your bed should be your source of liberation from the waking world. Make sure the feel and color of each component of your bed makes you *feel* good, adorning it with a comfortable mattress and luscious sheets both you and your partner love. If the person you sleep with is always complaining about the giant pink mandala in the center of your comforter, you won't go to bed in peace. Create your dream bed as a team!

- **Feng shui bed guidelines:** Your bed is a primary supporter of your energy, and it will nourish your whole being if it's put together in a way that resonates with you. The optimal "feng shui–approved" headboard is composed of solid wood that will literally and figuratively give your back and head good protection and support. Choose a wood you find beautiful and inviting. Place the headboard against a solid wall, making sure it's not blocking a window or preventing a door from being fully opened. Balance out bedroom energy by placing matching nightstands and lamps on either side of the bed, and try to avoid items with sharp edges.

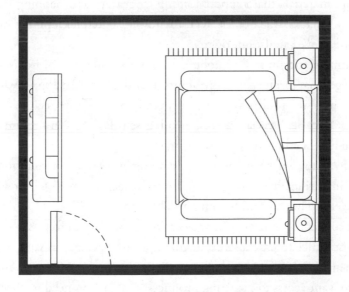

Example of optimal bed placement

- **Dressing:** If possible, consolidate all of your dressing needs in one area, and organize them in order of use, so your dressing ritual flows. For example, exercise clothing, then undergarments, then tops, then bottoms, then dresses, then pajamas. Store your shoes and accessories near where you usually put them on (i.e., bathroom or hallway closet). There's no need to strictly follow these organization suggestions, but do use categories and sorting methods that make sense to your lifestyle — and keep it *simple*.

- **Creativity:** This is the space where you play in your mind, exploring worlds created by others with words, cleaning out your brain with your pen and journal, or letting your spirit wander while looking out the window. In your early days of baby lovin' your creativity nook may double as your baby soothing and feeding zone, but when Baby is older, I recommend you keep this space for your tush only. You need a space that is just for you, free of spit-up and colorful plastic. Set up this space next to a source of natural light, and include a special chair and storage area that allows you to stash your inspirational materials. While you're sharing the space with Baby, store materials that support feeding, soothing, and napping (e.g., mama snacks, water bottle, teething toys, blanket, neck pillow, masseuse... We can dream, right?).

- **Intimate stimulus:** This nook is more of a collection of items and images that inspire an energy of intimacy than an actual space where you have sex (unless you have a special chair?). Store scented candles, lingerie, "special" books, or other sensual items in this area so you have a go-to source of sex-spiration.

- **Baby:** Baby will have a nook in just about every room of your home. By intentionally creating a baby zone in each room, you'll prevent the entire home from becoming Baby's domain. Whether you plan on cosleeping or having Babe sleep in her own room from the start, it's still nice to have a safe and cozy spot to place her in your room when it's time for nap, bath, or potty time...for Mommy. You'll also want access to diapering products stat. All you need to create a makeshift changing station is a contoured changing pad or mat and a diaper caddy with the essentials — wipes, baby booty cream, a few changes of clothes, and a baby distracter. Oh, and diapers.

- **Electronics:** Because digi-stalking your baby-less friends or watching a marathon of rich women arguing over seating arrangements at a dinner party can be strangely addictive, I recommend limiting electronics in the bedroom. But hey, movies in bed on a rainy day are pretty amazing, so place an aesthetically pleasing screen or barrier in front of your television when it's not in use and bring your phone or computer into the bedroom only when it's desperately needed — like when you're in bed nursing and you need to text your partner to ask them to bring you a batch of sweet potato fries and a Popsicle. Emergencies happen.

Leave It Out

For the sake of your serenity (and mental health) just say no to the following "visual to-dos" in the bedroom:

- **Anything related to work:** This is a no-brainer. And if your partner is your coworker, make them sleep on the couch! Just kidding — we love you, Partner! (Of course, your partner is a "visual to-do" in another sense…)
- **Exercise equipment:** You do not need to be thinking about reps when you're trying to get to REM. If your only storage option for exercise equipment is your bedroom, cover it with a shoji screen when it's not in use.
- **Cleaning supplies:** No. Just no.
- **An actual to-do list.**
- **"Maybe?" clutter:** If you're still holding on to a few "maybe" items, get rid of them, Girl.

Furniture Placement

Pretend you opened your bedroom door and water flowed into it. Would the water stagnate in a certain area, or would it be able to move freely? Stagnant energy, often caused by ill-placed furniture, can make your room feel heavy. To avoid this, ensure no piece of furniture is bursting the bubble of another piece of furniture, or preventing a door or drawer from fully opening — everyone needs their own space.

If you plan to add or replace furniture, measure your bedroom and draw a simple floor plan, confirming that the new pieces you're moving in will easily fit. Doing so will save you from frustration and preserve your relationships with friends or family members who gave up their Saturday to help you move furniture. (And you shouldn't be moving furniture! You're pregnant — sit in a chair and direct everyone.)

When organizing furniture, make sure the most appealing piece of furniture is the focal point when you enter. If the sight of your bed or your "snuggle chair" fills you with a sense of serenity, place it in a prominent location.

Maintain the Simplicity

- **Make your bed!** This is the easiest way to refresh the calm vibes in your bedroom. And it's unsatisfying to climb into an unmade bed at the end of a long day.
- **Daily five-minute put-away:** Take five minutes (or less) to put away items in your bedroom that have taken a temporary vacation from their assigned homes. You'll end your day with an organized space, saving you from the stress of waking up to visual "put-me-aways!" (Of course, you'll still be waking up to your little "pick-me-up"!)
- **Don't forget to donate:** Place an out-of-sight donation bag or box in your bedroom or closet. When you see an item that is no longer useful or has ceased to make you happy, put it in your donation bin. When the bin is full, take it to your chosen recipient of no-longer-needed goods. Don't look through the bin before you donate it — no second-guessing your initial decision! Your gut instinct is rarely wrong.
- **Three-month throw-away:** Every few months, give your bedroom some TLC via purging. Purging can mean throwing yuck stuff in the trash, putting cool but unneeded belongings in the donation pile, and scrapping organizing systems that are no longer working, replacing them with simple systems that suit your ever-evolving needs. Purging only once a year is the fuse that can lead to a panic attack.

Once you've kissed your bedroom with simplicity, soak in the results of your exerted energy. Sit in that chair or lie on that yummy-smelling bedding and *feel* the fresh and calm vibes in the space. Allow the energy of this sanctuary to fill you with a deep knowing that whatever flavors of challenge pregnancy and motherhood feed you, you'll always have this safe and healing nest to return to.

RIDDLE: What should be emitted from three different sources and levels in every room to evoke a nurturing energy?

Go to **YourSereneLife.wordpress.com/chapter-fourteen** and use the one-word riddle answer as your offer code to download the relaxation recording for this chapter.

CALL TO PLEASURE

* Lovingly evict all clutter from your bedroom.
* Fill your bedroom with soothing colors and fresh air.
* Create "energy nooks" by designating particular areas of your room for specific activities that evoke unique blends of energy.
* Invite the following treats into your bedroom:

  o Bedding you *love*
  o Three to five of your favorite images (hung in beautiful frames) that inspire romance and relaxation
  o Matching nightstands and lamps
  o One floor lamp near a reading chair
  o Baby nook items: bedside sleeper (or any other safe location where baby can sleep), changing pad, and stocked diaper caddy including diapers, wipes, baby-distracter, and change of clothes
  o Additional storage, if needed: baskets, bins, and boxes you love to look at
  o Silk screens, if needed, to cover television or exercise equipment
  o Reading chair, if you have the space
  o *And nothing else!* Just kidding. But do keep the other stuff to a minimum.

* Ask yourself, "How does this space make me *feel*?" If anything seems off, trust your instincts and change it.

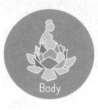

CHAPTER FIFTEEN

THE JOURNEY OF BIRTHING:
Phases of Labor

JUST BREATHE: *Envision liquid morphine being poured into a hollow in your mind. Each time you take a deep-in-the-belly breath, allow a bit of the "mind morphine" to flow out of the hollow and enter your bloodstream. The deeper your breath, and the higher your belly rises, the more mind-morphine is released, and the more euphoric you feel.*

Birth makes a biological imprint on you and your baby. Your cells, and those of your baby, remember birth and infuse the impact of this memory into various aspects of your lives. So yeah, your birth experience is important. You can create a more positive birth imprint by removing a few slices of the unknown from the birth experience.

Dread of the unknown is a powerful energy that can wreak havoc on the psyche. The actual birthing experience is the ultimate unknown for all women — even women who have given birth before. While reading this chapter you will learn that although birthing can be unpredictable, there are common stages and milestones you can expect and rely on. Allow yourself to be put at ease as you read about the common physiological and psychological experiences you will likely encounter during birth. In this chapter and the next, you will learn effective strategies for soothing yourself and managing any discomfort that accompanies the primary stages of labor and birth. You will come away from this chapter and the next with a clear plan for how to maintain peace, comfort, and excitement throughout the physical challenges and pivotal moments of childbirth.

What Is Labor?

Labor is defined as the period from the time your cervix begins to open and thin until the moment your placenta emerges. It's a time warp of beautiful chaos. Though there are common phases to labor — early labor, active labor, transition, birthing baby, and birthing the placenta — there are no set time limits on these phases. So it's best to focus more on the physical sensations your body is experiencing, rather than how much time has passed. You may blast through early labor in two hours, or watch a *Scandal* marathon before your body decides to eke into active labor — there is no "right or wrong" timing for labor, so just let it unfold.

While the phases of labor seem clear on paper, their lines are very fuzzy when applied to real life. It's unlikely you'll be aware of the exact moment you shift from early to active labor, or active labor to transition. The clearest information you'll receive in regard to where you are on the labor map is the number your cervix is dilated to (from 1 cm to 10 cm), and the position of your baby's head in your pelvis, called the *station* (ranging from –3 to +3; see image below).

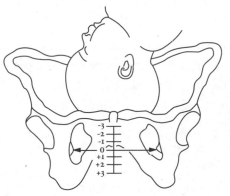

These numbers indicate the position of Baby's head in your pelvis during descent. You'll likely hear your care provider use these numbers as they track your progress through labor.

While these numbers can tell you how wide your cervix is yawning and how engaged your baby's head is, they're not crystal balls. You could sit pretty (hopefully not puke-y) at 5 cm and +1 for four hours, or you could fly from 6 cm and −1 to 10 cm and "pushing!" in a matter of minutes. No crystal balls, just predictably unpredictable labor.

Fortunately, there are milestones that commonly accompany each phase of labor, and ways to make them more comfortable. Here they are.

Early Labor

The earliest phase of labor, when the cervix gradually opens and thins, often lasts the longest but is the least intense. This opening and thinning is supported by relaxin, a hormone secreted by the placenta, that has also been softening the ligaments in your pelvis. If this phase begins days before your baby is ready to emerge, you may not even notice the surges that accompany it.

When your baby triggers the "green light" you'll likely notice most of your surges but will be able to talk through them. These surges will last thirty to forty-five seconds and may be irregular, possibly twenty minutes (or more) apart. This phase causes you to feel some gentle tugs and tightening, and maybe extra loose bowel movements. (I keep using words like *possibly* and *maybe* because birth doesn't fit into a predetermined box.)

During early labor your cervix will progress to 3–4 cm, and you'll *probably* experience a few of these symptoms:

- Release of membranes (water breaking). This may be in a gush, like in the movies, or in an "I'm slowing wetting myself" trickle. Check to make sure the water does not have a foul odor or discoloration.
- Vaginal mucus tinged with blood (just as delectable as it sounds)
- Diarrhea!
- Pressure in the lower abdomen
- Period-like cramps
- Pressure or tightening in the lower back
- Heartburn
- A feeling of excitement, confusion, anxiety, relief, or all of the above — at once

- An overwhelming desire to scrub the grout in your shower or organize your bathing suit drawer

What to Do

- **Sleep:** It will likely be the last thing you feel like doing when you go into labor, but get some rest. One of the most common complaints I hear from moms in the later stages of labor is that they're exhausted. Sure, the physical act of labor can be anywhere from a little to extremely tiring, but it doesn't help that many women haven't slept for over twenty-four hours by the time Baby pokes his head out. At least pretend to take a nap.
- **Distract yourself:** Waiting for early labor to kick up a notch can be like waiting for work to be over on a Monday. If you can't sleep, go for a walk (take your cell phone!), watch a movie, cook some food, fold some tiny clothes, scrub that grout, or do anything else that distracts you from watching the proverbial water boil.
- **Eat something:** Just as with the sleep issue, many women groan into the last phase of labor, depleted because they haven't eaten since… "I had some crackers about sixteen hours ago." Get some nourishment down your gullet, preferably something protein rich (not fat and sugar rich) that will sustain you through a marathon.
- **Tell your partner:** If your partner is not with you, you don't need to call a police escort to get them to you *now*, but you should gently alert them that something is happening. They can then alert their boss that they may need to leave early, tell their drinking buddy to call an Uber, or have a panic attack before their energy mixes with yours.
- **Just breathe:** Practice your deep breathing so intently it becomes second nature by the time your body is *really* in need of focused breath work.
- **Nourish your bladder:** Don't become so excited about Baby coming that you forget to pee. A full bladder can impede Baby's descent, and Baby's descent can impede your ability to pee, so empty that sucker out as much as possible before it forgets how to #LetItGo.

Call Your Care Provider Immediately, If...

If your membranes release and the water has a green tinge, if you have bright-red discharge, if you don't feel your baby moving, or if you just have an overwhelming urge to let your care provider know what's happening, call them. None of these circumstances warrant a freak-out; they're just important pieces of information for your care provider to be privy to.

What Not to Do

- **Rush to the birth center or hospital, or call in the tribe:** Don't up jump tha boogie and get everyone geared up for birth prematurely. Enjoy the gentleness of this early phase of labor by spending quiet time with your Self, or your partner. This is the last time your life will be in this state — relish it. Having "your people" start to exert energy before it's needed will poop them out before you really need them to keep their poop together!

Active Labor

This period can last anywhere from twenty-ish minutes to many-ish hours, but it's usually shorter than early labor. You'll progress to 7–8 cm during this time, and surges will likely be stronger and closer together (usually three to four minutes apart) and have a more distinctive "peak." You'll feel pressure beginning to pool in your nether regions; bloody mucus, and water if your membranes have not yet released, may journey out of your vagina; and fatigue may replace the initial gusto you had for birth.

If you're in a hospital or birth center, your doula and companion will be offering psychological and physiological support (maybe rubbing your back and telling you that you make childbirth look sexy), while the medical care providers will be staying out of your way, only intermittently checking your blood pressure and monitoring the strength and length of your surges and Baby's heart rate.

If you were watching a movie or playing Scrabble during early labor, you've now written off the plot or started using four-letter words on the board. This phase of labor demands more of you — *all* of you. This doesn't have to be a negative experience. The intensity can serve to help you travel further within and partially dissociate your mind from the physical sensations of your body, or begin to process them as something separate from pain.

I really despised the early phase of my labor as I got used to the foreign sensations of my birth. But by the time I reached active labor, I was so used to the sensations that I was able to check my mind out of the penitentiary of pain. Part of my mind stayed in my body to be aware of what it needed (deep breathing and good posture), but the other hunk floated to this watery space above my body, where I saw myself riding black waves.

What to Do

You may hit a wall at the beginning of this phase as you figure out how to process the more intense sensations. Try these practices to settle into this heightened level of labor:

- **Put your people to work:** While you might have been cool about processing your birthing sensations on your own in early labor, you'll need to wake up your tribe when you enter active labor. You may not know what you need or want, and will rely on them to lead you into various techniques that will make you more comfortable and help you settle. If you have a doula, they'll already know to make the suggestions below. If you're going at it without a professional emotional supporter, make a copy of these suggestions for your birth companion to rely on during this phase.
- **Shift your body:** Just keep trying different positions; maybe sit in the tub or shower, squat on the floor, lay on your other side, do some yoga, get out a Kama Sutra book, whatever — just move your body until you notice some relief. When you've found the savory spot you'll likely notice that it's easier to deeply inhale and exhale through your nose. Settle into this space and allow your mind to float away. Make another move when your breath work becomes difficult, or your body tightens.
- **Regulate your temperature:** You may notice that waves of heat drift over you, or a case of the shivers seeps into you during this time.

If you're hot, ask for a wet washcloth for your forehead (with a few drops of your essential oil of choice — peppermint is cooling); or if you're chilly, a cozy blanket. Drink regular doses of water to manage your inner thermometer.

- **Eat:** If your energy is deserting you and you feel hungry, eat a light protein-rich snack.

- **Sit on the toilet:** Ideally, something will come out as you sit on the toilet. Because it will become increasingly difficult to relieve your bladder or bowels the deeper you move into labor, now is a great time to do it. Beyond that goal, sitting on the toilet gives your body the signal to open and release, often helping to bolster labor. So in between surges, put all your concentration on letting it flow.

What Not to Do

- **Be talked into something you're not okay with:** This is often the time when certain people suggest interventions to "speed things along" or "make you more comfortable." If you spend time marinating on these options and intuitively feel good about one or all of them, go for it. But don't allow yourself to be pressured into something you'll later regret. Ask as many questions as you can think of if an intervention is recommended, the first being, "Is this a medical emergency? Does my well-being or that of my baby heavily rely on this intervention?" If the answers are "No," you have more time to consider your options. Ask about alternative options, and see if everyone can leave you alone for a while so you can discuss it with your birth companion. Or, just politely decline. Do you, Mama.

Transition

Whoa, Nelly — here we go!

Transition is exciting! And overwhelming. Your cervix is fully dilating to 10 cm and your baby's head is likely fully engaged in the pelvic region. This phase often lasts the shortest amount of time and is the most intense. Welcome to the tipping point, when you have a spiritual awakening, momentarily beg for an epidural, assault anyone who enters the room with pleas to help you escape, or have a rolling orgasm. Anything goes during transition. It will likely include the most intense surges you've had thus far, and while I feel like a jerk writing this, these surges are a good sign. They mean your baby is making moves, and you're near the end and close to a new beginning. It's terrifying, and fabulous.

During this time you may be hit with all the things, all at once: a throbbing back, the urge to poop (without any poop), bloody vaginal discharge, hot-cold-hot-cold, shaky legs, an urge to vomit (or actual vomiting), and a soul-deep yearning to just take a nap. Oh, and excitement. Even though it may seem like your body is deciding whether it will implode or explode, all these happenings mean Baby is *close*. You're going to become a mama soon, and all this crazy-hard physical stuff will subside.

What to Do

- **Ride the waves:** Just let it happen — all you need to do is let it happen. When you surrender to the all-consuming sensations that gush through you during transition, it passes more quickly. When this phase is met with space and acceptance (rather than constrictive resistance), it finishes its work of opening you to 10 cm and then steps aside to allow you to start doing the strangely pleasing work of pushing, or breathing, your baby down.

- **Focus on your mega-level of awesomeness:** You've come *so* far. You successfully conceived (maybe with the help of IVF doctors — even cooler!), grew that baby into a fully formed being, went through two stages of not-easy labor, and you're Here! Your world is about to be bust open by the most delicious sounds of newborn wails, love that will make you dizzy, and the delivery of the best meal that's ever passed through your lips. Life is good — well, almost. Just keep going!

- **Hang on to that breath work like a lifeline:** Because transition puts a bit of force on your body (the understatement to end all understatements), you need to ensure you're getting oxygen to your baby. Deep breaths will help to regulate Baby's heart rate during this time, and getting that oxygen to her little body could make the difference between strongly encouraged interventions and accolades. Breathe, Mama, just breathe.

- **Tell them to get their hands off you, or to stop talking:** The gentle massage and soothing affirmations your supporters have been providing up to this point may now feel like anguish. If you don't want any of it, speak up! You're not being rude, you're in labor. If you haven't been receiving that physical and verbal assistance, but now feel that it will help, speak up! Ask for what you need, or at least what you think you need.

What Not to Do

- **Expect your baby any moment:** Being fully dilated is a huge milestone, very stoke-worthy. But there's still some work ahead. If you've already had a vaginal birth, you may be one of those "three pushes and he was out!" ladies, but if your vagina and all its friends are novices at this, the pushing may take a while. Set the intention that you will be filled with a mega-recharge of energy and determination after you've moved through transition.

Birthing Baby

You've been fully dilated for ages! You're ready to push! But wait. Your surges stopped? What's going on?

You may have entered the very common resting phase where your surges slow, or completely stop, for a period of time. If you and your baby are healthy, this rest is no cause for alarm; it's a wonderful chance for you to doze and refuel before the most labor-intense (hehe) portion of childbirth begins. I recommend you take a nap, eat a little food, and drink water. Then, give a little love to your nipples. Nipple stimulation can trigger the release of oxytocin and turn your inner wave machine back on.

What to Do

Your surges turned back on? Care provider said it's time to bear down, or breathe down? *You* feel the urge to bear or breathe down? Yay! Move forward into this final phase, Mama Grasshopper — you are ready.

- **Act only during surges:** Throughout each surge during this time, you will be prompted by your supporters (hopefully in strong and direct, yet peaceful tones) to bear down (like you're having a bowel movement) or breathe down (like you're sending a powerful breath down the back of your throat, through your uterus, and out your vagina). You will likely be able to do a few pushes, or birth breaths, with each surge. Then, between surges, close your eyes, go totally limp, and breathe normally. (The difference between "bearing down" and "breathing down" is explained further on page 211.) Envision each breath refilling you with energy and power, recharging you for the next surge.

- **Change positions:** Ask for help shifting positions after each round of four or five surges until you settle into the position you and your supporters feel is most effective. This shifting may also give baby the slight repositioning she needs to settle into the optimal position for emergence.

- **Surrender to the fullness, amnesia, and time distortion:** This phase will magnify the sensation of fullness so intensely that you may feel natural numbness in your perineum. You'll be so focused on your mission that you'll probably forget much of what is said or done. And the ecstatic hormones rushing through you may cause you to be oblivious to time. I found these experiences really pleasing, but some women find them overwhelming. I bring them up because I want you to know that nothing is wrong if you experience these "otherworldly," sometimes psychedelic-like sensations; you're just having a baby.

- **Request a perineal massage:** This involves your care provider rubbing natural oil around your perineum to soften and "slick it up" for Baby's emergence. Most care providers will do this of their own volition, but it's nice to be forewarned about their beneficial vaginal meddling. They'll likely start this ritual when Baby's head is crowning, or being so close to emerging that you can reach down and feel the top of his head!

- **Expect emotional explosions!** When your baby *finally* emerges, you will be overcome with joy, confusion, relief, concern, urging, purging, and everything in between. Let it come. You just emerged, just like your baby. You were just born as a mother, and your baby was just born as her own being — soon to be separated from your physical body. This will also be the first time you experience the sensation of a piece of your soul existing outside your body — it's like your baby claimed a little piece of it while she lived in your womb.

- **Know that it's normal if you *don't* feel the explosions:** Some women take a while to "get there" — sometimes months, and that's okay. Your body (and mind, and soul) just went through an epic journey, throwing up chaotic hormones all over the path. You may feel totally depleted, even a little sad and disconnected. This does not mean that you're a bad mother, or that you'll never feel that loving infatuation for your child. But it does mean you should let someone know how you're feeling. Postpartum blues, or postpartum depression, is no longer taboo or ignored; it's finally being acknowledged as an organic phase in the experience of many mothers. Tell your care provider how you're feeling so they can work to get you support in the form of counseling, extra postpartum assistance, or in more serious situations, medications to help your hormones chill out. And remember, you're still a rockstar-warrior-mama!

- **Get to bonding:** Even if you're having trouble feeling that initial surge of euphoria, start going through the motions of bonding; they just might lift that initial fog. Have your baby placed on your bare chest as soon as possible, with a blanket covering his back for warmth but not coming between your bodies. This skin-to-skin will help baby regulate his breathing, heart rate, blood pressure, and temperature and will help soothe him after the adventure of birth. Speak or sing softly to him, gazing into his eyes, and cradle his smooth, tiny body. If he starts bobbing his head around your chest and you feel ready, ask for assistance to try out breastfeeding.

What Not to Do

- **Berate yourself:** Once your baby is born and you're free of the majority of birthing sensations, your mind will have space to take stock of how your birth went. If you feel an aspect of birth did not go as expected and you're unhappy with that, acknowledge it, breathe, and for the moment, move on. There will be time to process any negative elements present in your birth, and to release them via strategies we'll explore in later chapters. For now, cherish the fresh life you just delivered and allow yourself to feel pride, love, and relief. You're amazing — honor that.

Birthing the Placenta

You birthed a baby — now you get to birth an organ! Your body births the placenta so your uterus can begin contracting back to its pre-pregnancy size, and because it no longer has any use for a placenta. The emergence of the placenta is not just an interesting medical phenomenon; it symbolizes a passage of responsibility for Baby's care from your inner world to your outer world. A major shift is occurring in the way you'll continue to nourish your baby's development; care now becomes a more constant and conscious decision, quite different from the modus operandi of pregnancy — caring for yourself and knowing that is probably enough to keep Baby happy.

The placenta usually takes five to thirty minutes to emerge, and unless it's an emergency situation, your care provider will allow it to emerge without physical assistance. It is common for care providers to recommend you receive an injection of synthetic oxytocin at this time to ensure that your surges continue. Your care provider will likely monitor the progress of the placenta and your vaginal bleeding (which is normal), so don't be alarmed if people are still between your legs when Baby is on your chest. It's common for a medical care provider to knead your lower abdomen to encourage the uterus to shrink back down to size and minimize bleeding. The kneading is not the most comfortable sensation, but you just had a baby, so small potatoes.

What to Do

- **Breastfeed:** Breastfeeding helps to stimulate the uterine surges that will expel the placenta and shrink the uterus back to its average size.

When you sense your baby is ready, direct her toward an exposed nipple to see if she has any interest in latching on.

- **Saving it? Remind them:** If you plan to have the placenta encapsulated, put this request in your birth preferences and have your birth companion or doula remind the medical staff you would like the placenta saved. They usually do this by putting it on ice until the person who will perform the dehydration and encapsulation comes to retrieve it.
- **Check it out!** Sure, the placenta is gory at first sight, but its essence is extraordinary. You grew that organ in the past nine months! Cool! Take a look, take a picture, brag about how big and healthy your placenta is.
- **Know there will be blood:** A bloody vaginal discharge called *lochia* will keep on keepin' on for many days after delivery. Expecting the blood will make its appearance less jarring.

And Finally…

After all humans and organs have been birthed, it's time for your vaginal reconstruction! Just kidding. But this is the time when your vagina will receive some TLC: stitches if you had any perineal tears (yay!), cold compresses to minimize vaginal swelling (yum), and a fatty maxi pad to catch the bleeding (sexy). You'll be nursing your tender vagina almost as much as your newborn your first month postpartum, so please go into this time knowing it's not just okay but *essential* to take it easy.

From Her Heart to Yours

My early labor lasted two hours, active labor four hours, transition two hours, and pushing six hours. I didn't know how loose the "average time frames for phases of labor" were. I thought I had an undiagnosed birthing deficiency because my birth pattern was so irregular. I sat in shame over this, feeling that if I'd only squatted more, or praised more birthing deities, or breathed deeper, I would have followed "the pattern."

I found healing when I discovered how normal "irregular" labor was. Every woman I interrogated about birth had a different tale to tell, not one birth the same. Many of our birthing signs and symptoms could have been cousins, but the manner and timing they expressed themselves in made them sound like renegades. My challenge in reconciling with the uncertainty of birth has made me a better mom, because I can now roll with the uncertainty that exists in every hot second of motherhood.

—T. T., Eugene, Oregon

RIDDLE: I'm the bloody vaginal discharge women experience for many days postpartum. What's my name?

Go to **YourSereneLife.wordpress.com/chapter-fifteen** and use the one-word riddle answer as your offer code to download the relaxation recording for this chapter.

CALL TO PLEASURE

Envision yourself moving through each phase of labor in the manner that seems ideal to you by following these steps. (Even if your labor does not happen exactly as you envision, this practice will send you into birth feeling more at ease and optimistic, serving to create a more favorable experience.)

1. Find a quiet and comfortable space to relax in.
2. In your mind's eye, envision yourself in the few days preceding the onset of labor looking and feeling relaxed and excited, engaging in activities you enjoy, and bonding with your family and unborn baby.
3. Now, imagine yourself noticing the first signs of labor, being surprised by how well you're handling this shift and how peaceful you feel about the prospect of doing the dang thang.
4. Your labor is picking up, and you see yourself utilizing techniques to make you more comfortable during this active stage of labor. You have a knowing that your cervix is easily opening.

5. Transition is intense, but it serves as a type of spiritual experience, connecting you with your deepest powers. You move through it quickly, feeling like a total goddess, grounded on Earth but dancing in the heavens.

6. It's time for Baby to emerge! Your body begins bearing down when it has the uncontrollable urge to do so, and you're able to breathe through it all, expressing an innate knowledge of how to support your body.

7. Now, feel and see yourself holding your new baby in your arms. Feel his silken skin, smell his perfect scent, breathe that baby in and fill him with your love.

8. Hey! Check you out! You and your babe are breastfeeding like champs! Your colostrum is flowing out in the perfect amount, and Baby is sucking down that liquid gold.

9. Feel it, see it, believe it.

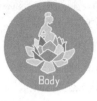

CHAPTER SIXTEEN

BIRTHING POSITIONS AND LIGHT TOUCH HEALING

JUST BREATHE. *Close your right nostril with your thumb, take a deep breath in, then release your right nostril while closing your left nostril with your pointer finger and slowly exhale. Repeat this cycle ten times. Put all of your attention into the tiny hairs in and around your nostrils, noticing how they feel as the air flows in and out.*

G iving birth on the moon would probably suck — gravity is lazy there. But gravity is active on Earth — a sacred gift to birthing mothers. So put it to use! In this chapter, I will discuss optimal (gravity-utilizing) birthing positions and their specific benefits, strategies to effectively communicate your positioning preferences to your care providers and team, and how your birthing companion can use massage and pressure points to heighten your comfort. You'll be urged to allow your body to surrender to its deep connection with nature and encouraged to develop trust in your body's ability to meet the awesome challenges of this experience with your unique expression of graceful power. (Howling? Dancing? Om-ing? Swirling? Cursing? It's all gravy, Baby.)

> HOUSEKEEPING: *If you have injuries or chronic conditions that restrict you from assuming certain positions, honor those circumstances and work with what your body can do.*

Discover What Positions Feel Good to You

Childbirth is not the time to force your body into contorted positions you've never tried before — pregnancy is the time to do this! Once a day, with the assistance of your birthing companion, practice one of the birthing positions outlined below. Be gentle with yourself, making adjustments as needed and taking a moment in each position to notice what you like and dislike about the orientation of your body. First, do a body scan from the top of your head to the tips of your toes, noticing how each nook and crevice of your body responds to the position. Then, go deeper into your inquiry by asking the following questions:

- How easily can I breathe in this position? (Readjust in the position until you find the sweet spot where your lungs can easily claim oxygen.)
- Do my legs feel strong in this position? If not, do I feel drawn to practice this position daily to build up my strength?
- Do I feel strained in this position? Do I need to utilize gentler stretching exercises to limber up before I move into birth?
- Does my pelvic region feel open and relaxed in this position? (Yes? This position could be your hero during birth, serving to widen the birth path and shorten labor.)
- Does this position connect me with the pull of gravity? (Do you feel a sensation of Baby being slightly pulled down in this position? Good.)
- Does this position make me feel emotionally and physically supported by my birth companion? (A position that creates an exchange of energy between you and your companion could serve to bolster your courage and determination during birth. If the position allows you to have a make-out session with your hun, even better; a relaxed kisser creates a relaxed vagina.)
- What *feels* good? If you hate the sensation of squatting, don't do it. Find what you like and keep doing that.

First *sample* the moves, then *practice* your favorites daily. And *tone* throughout, by regularly performing exercises that strengthen the muscles called on by your fave positions.

Stirrups

While the "flat on your back, feet up in stirrups" position generally gets a bad rap (because it can feel pretty awful and usually serves the needs of the medical staff more than the mother), it may still be your favorite. Don't discount any position just because of the lore surrounding it. If you try this position and find it comfortable and supportive of your birthing needs, stick with it! But if your care provider keeps placing you in that position and it all feels wrong, change it up. You are not legally obligated to stay in any position. If you select this position on your own, I encourage you to make it less supine by elevating your back and head with a few pillows.

Squatting

Squatting is a position utilized daily in many cultures (e.g., Chinese, Southeast Asian, and Eastern European) for cooking, cleaning, sex, and…birthing. Squatting facilitates a surrender to gravity and opens the door for Baby to emerge. But it is not a common position for women in most developed countries. (If sitting in an office chair or the bucket seat of a car in traffic were optimal positions for birthing, we'd be golden.) With the support of your partner, ease into the following positions with the knowing that it may take some time for you to become fully comfortable in a squat. Slight stretching and mild exertion of your muscles is normal, but if you experience any pain, ease out of the position.

LEAPFROG SQUAT

This is the richest form of squatting. If you plan to utilize this position during birth, have your companion lower you into it daily and see if you feel most comfortable supporting your weight by placing your hands on the floor in front of you, or behind you. If you're very comfortable in a low squat, you can practice with your hands in prayer position, as shown. This low squat can increase the rotation of

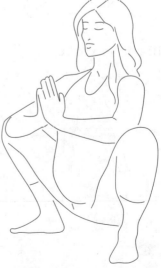

Baby, improve fetal circulation, and widen the diameter of your pelvis (up to 2 cm!), and it requires less "pushing" effort from you.

Supported squat

If you feel too tenuous supporting your own weight, have your birth companion sit on a chair behind you, supporting your weight by placing their arms under your armpits.

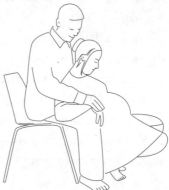

Standing squat

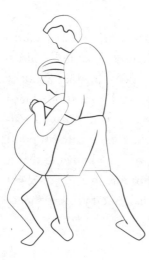

The idea of going all the way with a squat may be laughable to you during surges. If so, have your partner stand with their legs in a wide stance and their arms extended out at the elbows. Slightly bend your knees and lean back into your companion's arms so they're supporting most of your weight. If movement feels good to you, your companion can gently sway you back and forth. This position also lengthens your torso, which can help Baby properly align with your pelvis. Have your companion lean their back against a wall if their balance feels unsteady.

Birthing stool

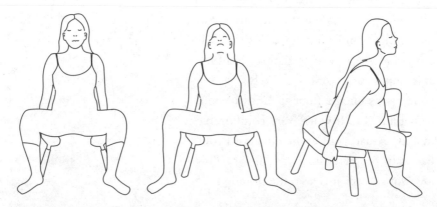

These horseshoe-shaped stools allow you to assume a deep squat without having to ask your legs for much effort. Because these stools provide good access to all things vagina, most care providers won't make a fuss if you want to birth your baby here.

Alternate Positions

Squatting is not the only way; here are alternate positions to try.

FORWARD LEAN

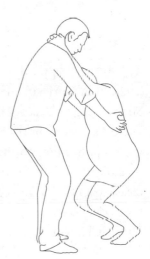

This can be a divine pose if you're having trouble maintaining a steady breathing pattern and prefer to have your weight leaning forward, rather than the backward leaning that tends to occur while squatting. Lay your head on your partner's shoulder or chest, with your arms wrapped around their neck or waist, and slightly bend your knees. Have your partner place their hands wherever you prefer; they can lightly run their fingers along your scalp or spine to stimulate the release of endorphins. Have them do a slow and deep breathing pattern through their nose, and work to match their depth and pace.

PILLOW NESTING

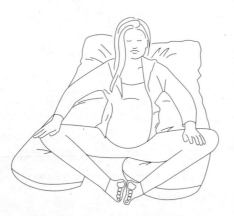

If you can't be bothered to exert any muscle but your uterus during birth, you can settle into a nest of pillows, ensuring your back is comfortably elevated so you're still tapping into gravity. This can be a helpful position if you're utilizing more mental than physical techniques during birth. If your body is able to go completely limp, it's easier for your mind to wander away.

SIDE LIE

This is the sleepy lady's pose. If everything down to your nose hair is exhausted, lie on your side so you can drift into quasi-sleep between surges. Sleep during labor is not the REM sleep you normally experience — it's more like a lucid twilight-zone sleep, but better than nothing. Allow yourself to go completely limp in this position when you're not surging. If you're in the final phase of labor, someone will help you lift your upper leg during surges to create space for Baby to come out. This position can help get oxygen to Baby, lower elevated blood pressure, improve the strength of surges, and help your birth chill if it's on the speed train (plus it works fine with an epidural).

HANDS AND KNEES

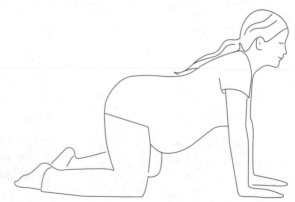

Is Baby in a funny position? Get on your hands and knees on a soft surface and swirl those hips. Or lay your head down on your arms, keep your butt in the air, and swirl your hips some more. These positions and movements can create the space and momentum to encourage your baby to get in the ideal position for birth, and they relieve back pain.

Speaking of the ideal position for Baby during birth...this figure shows where you want Baby to be.

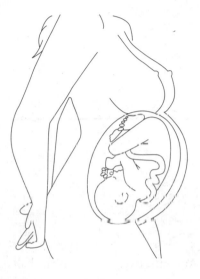

TOILET

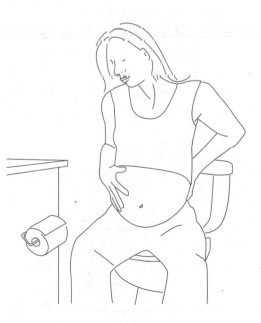

Your body is used to opening and releasing on the toilet, and this reaction is no different during birth. If you're in a birth center or hospital, chances are there will be a support bar by the toilet you can lean on. And don't worry — when your baby's head is about to emerge, your helpers will have you shift positions so the baby doesn't fall into the toilet. If the pressure from the toilet seat is uncomfortable, ask for a donut cushion.

Birth ball

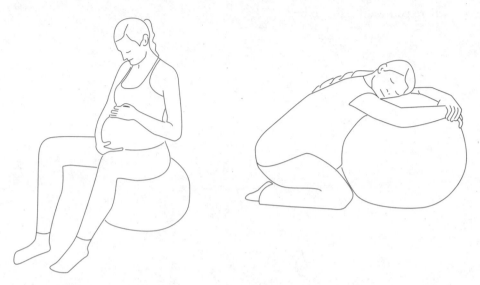

Birth balls are fun. And effective. Sit on a birth ball and lean forward onto a bed or your partner, or place your knees on a pillow on the floor and lean onto the birth ball. The ball facilitates a fluid movement in the hips, which helps to keep any stagnant energy spiraling down and out of you, potentially speeding up the birth process and minimizing your discomfort. When you're sitting on the ball, pressure is taken off your hips and your pelvic region relaxes. When you're leaning on it, your back is free to welcome a light touch massage, hip squeeze, or pressure point work.

Tub or shower

If in doubt, get in some warm water, Woman.

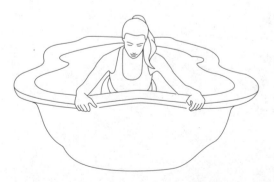

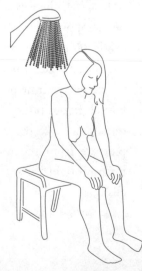

Swirl into Your Strength

Making circular movements during experiences that are otherwise usually processed as painful sends signals to receptors in your brain to minimize their perception of pain. Swirling is the most organic movement you can flow into during surges, and it helps pain funnel down and out, being replaced by a rush of endorphins. These circular motions also help Baby progress downward. If you feel lingering tension after a surge, continue the swirling until the tightness has loosened. Prenatal hip swirls also strengthen your abdominal wall, serving to minimize chances of diastasis recti (abdominal separation), reduce back pain, and make your surges more effective.

Stretching

A runner stretches before and after a marathon, right? Well, each surge is like a mini-marathon, so you may need to stretch your muscles in between. No need to get all Gumby with it, just get the blood reflowing through your muscles by stretching your arms above your head, pointing and flexing your feet, or doing any other stretch that feels good and easy to you.

Touch

Your energy alone may not be enough to get you through childbirth. The energy of others, transmitted through touch during birth, could support you in releasing tension in freaked-out muscles, encourage your nervous system and pituitary glands to start pumping out endorphins, and get you past the urge to scream for an epidural. (On the other hand, if touch during labor makes you want to punch someone, ask them to stop.)

The type of touch you'll respond to throughout birth will shift, depending on the phase of labor you're in and how your body is processing it. Practice the following methods with your birth companion so you're both familiar with what feels good to you when you eventually move into childbirth, keeping in mind that what feels good to you now may feel very different when your body is in labor.

- **Light touch massage:** When you gently graze the back of your fingertips across your skin, endorphins are released, relaxation is sparked, and stagnant energy in your body is released. You can practice light touch massage on yourself (I do it on my forearm when I'm in the car and have to pee!), but to access the back, which is the area that will likely require the most attention during birth, you'll want your birth companion to get those fingertips ready. To keep the strokes fluid, ask them to start with the back of their fingertips at the base of your spine, then have them swirl the back of their fingers up your back in a figure eight pattern. They can then continue down your arms, then up your neck and scalp. When they're done with one cycle, have them return their fingers to the base of your spine and repeat as many times as you like.

- **Pressure points:** Applying pressure to the end points of certain meridians, or pathways in the body where vital energy flows, can help to reduce discomfort during labor (or at any time!). The following images show various points that you or your companion can apply pressure to during labor. Some may feel wonderful; some may feel like torture. Guide your companion, telling them what points feel good and how much pressure you require. If you desire deeper pressure, you can ask your companion to use their thumbs, knuckles, elbows, or even a tennis ball to get all up in there.

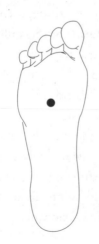

This point is located in the depression that appears in the upper middle portion of the sole of the foot when it is flexed. Applying pressure to this point may reduce anxiety, dizziness, headaches, neck pain, and nausea.

These points are located on the shoulders halfway between the rotator cuffs and spine. Applying pressure to these points reduces discomfort in the neck and shoulders, and may facilitate the release of the placenta after birth.

These points are located at the base of the skull in the indentations on both sides of the neck. Applying pressure to these points releases endorphins, alleviates discomfort in the head and pressure in the eyes, and increases energy levels.

These points are located in the dimple of the buttocks, usually found one to two inches away from both sides of the base of the spine. Applying pressure to these points may induce labor and reduce discomfort in the lower back.

This point is located on the outside of the foot between the Achilles tendon and anklebone. Applying pressure to this point may induce labor, reduce pain in the lower back, and bring more general comfort to a difficult labor.

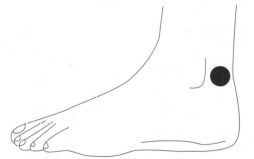

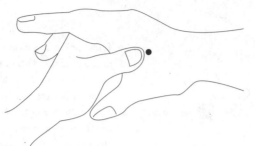

This point is located between the web of the thumb and pointer finger at the highest point of the muscle. Applying pressure to this point may induce labor, reduce overall labor discomfort, and relieve headaches.

- **Hip squeeze:** Because your hips are hit with a Mack Truck of pressure during birth, applying pressure to this area can push things back into a relaxed state, offering you one of the tastiest flavors of relief. This pressure can also encourage your baby to get moving down and out. Give your partner access to your back, preferably by leaning forward onto a bed or birth ball. Next, have them place their palms on the fleshy part of each side of your hips, with their fingertips facing each other and hands parallel to the ground. Now, they should apply pressure down and in, like they were trying to squeeze your butt cheeks together! Yay! Have them toy around with hand positioning and pressure until a resounding "yes!" releases within you.

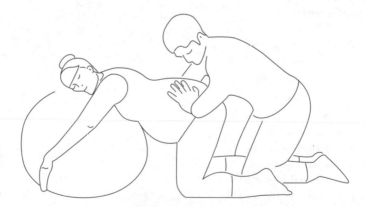

Through each phase of birth, cycle through these methods until you settle on the one that feels best at the time, which may be no touch at all. When that choice no longer feels good, try something else. For methods that require more effort from your companion (like hip pressure), encourage them to use their whole body, instead of just their arms, and to be cognizant of properly positioning their body so they can sustain this support. If possible, have them periodically switch off with another birth supporter so they can recharge.

Science Says...

Smart people at the Touch Research Institute reported that birthing women whose partners massaged them felt less depressed, had less labor pain, and had lower stress and anxiety levels. They found that the physical involvement of a partner corresponded to less need for pain medication, shorter labors, fewer complications, and happier mamas. And not all touch is equal — another study found that moms found massage administered by a partner or doula more therapeutic than touch given by a medical care provider.

Keep 'Em Busy

One of the greatest benefits to all this "touchy feely" is that it keeps your partner occupied. Birth companions can become anxious when they can't do anything to help, and this nervous energy reverberates into you. Keep them busy touching you (or walking laps around the parking lot if they're stressing you out). Because practice makes adeptness, take advantage of this brief fissure in time when you can justify a request for a massage as necessary preparation for childbirth.

Do What Feels Good

If you find a position, pressure point, voodoo witch doctor chant, wheatgrass elixir, or anything else that is not on this list but feels good (and is safe) — do it. No one will know exactly how your mind-body-spirit will respond to labor until you're actually in labor. So take all these suggestions, stick them in your goody bag, and pull them out if they sound good during birth, or use them to inspire a new form of relief. Just keep trying different strategies until you find that burst of solace, and when that burst fizzles, shift into a new strategy, allowing your body to lead the charge.

From Her Heart to Yours

I was more flexible and fit after having a baby. Before pregnancy I hated stretching and thought my friends who swore by yoga were super lame. Practicing birth positions and realizing how stiff I was forced me to begin stretching, and even order a prenatal yoga DVD. The process of limbering my body for birth heightened my willingness to be more adventurous, not just in body, but in mind and spirit as well. As I began to feel the benefits of the stretching and saw how well they improved my ability to "do birth well," I began exploring other "expansive" options I used to think of as "super lame" — like meditating. Thanks, birthing positions, for making me better at life.

— *A. M., Los Angeles, California*

RIDDLE: What position can expand the diameter of your cervix by up to two centimeters?

Go to **YourSereneLife.wordpress.com/chapter-sixteen** and use the one-word riddle answer as your offer code to download the relaxation recording for this chapter.

CALL TO PLEASURE

- Practice birthing positions with your partner to facilitate toning and bonding.
- Decide what positions feel best and practice them daily.
- Practice intentional breathing while in your favorite positions.
- Practice touch techniques with your partner to alleviate pregnancy discomforts.

CHAPTER SEVENTEEN

HOW TO BREATHE

JUST BREATHE: *Take in ten slow and steady breaths of gratitude, meditating on how amazing it is to have an abundance of life-giving energy constantly willing to flow into you, to pull toxins out of you.*

The breath is the surest path to serenity. Focused breathing fills you and your baby with the substance of life, supports the uterus in its birthing efforts, and allows you to float into an intentional state of calm. This chapter will instill in you a desire to make purposeful breathing a constant in your life as you learn the multitude of benefits conscious breathing holds, and develop a deeper connection to the spiritual nature of your breath work. While breathing is an involuntary act of your body, your mind can choose to place intention into the act, creating a powerful mind-body bridge.

A neat thing about focused breathing is you can practice it while scrambling eggs, vacuuming, or changing a diaper (there's a really bizarre primal pleasure in smelling your newborn's soiled diaper essence...). Sitting quietly and meditating on your breath is beneficial, but you don't have to wait for a quiet moment to utilize this peace-inducing practice. You can do it now. No really, do it now.

The Importance of Oxygen

So first there's that thing about not being able to survive more than a few minutes without it. Obviously we need oxygen. But beyond that, the intake of this element releases toxins, soothes stress, brings clarity of mind, makes you happier, helps to maintain muscle health, keeps your figure sexy, improves your posture... *and* pleases your baby. In addition, conscious breathing connects you to something deeper than your physical experience; it allows you to pull grounding energy from the Earth and sinks you into the juicy core of each moment, which is where introspection and gratitude live. As we continue to explore the benefits of deep breathing I want you to notice any mental, physical, or emotional shifts you feel.

Toxin Release

Your body is a first-rate toxin killer, releasing those poisons every chance it gets. Depriving your body of toxin-releasing breaths is like forgetting to roll your trash bin to the curb every Sunday. If your body is left with a buildup of toxins, your organs are required to work overtime to flush out the yuck. Guess what happens when your organs get burnt out? They get sick and have shortened life spans.

One of these toxic offenders is carbon dioxide. Too much carbon dioxide in your blood can cause central nervous system damage, respiratory function deterioration, low blood pressure, cardiac arrhythmia, and asphyxiation. On a less gnarly scale, it can cause fatigue, shortness of breath, confusion, headaches, and constipation — that's right, breathing helps you poop.

What prevents cancer? Your white blood cells detecting and eliminating unwanted mutant cells. When the body is not supplied with enough oxygen to flush out bodily toxins, our white blood cells begin to perish, leaving the body more susceptible to disease.

And did you know one pint of blood is pumped through the uterus every minute of your pregnancy, gifting the placenta with nutrients? This pumping diminishes if you're not pulling in enough oxygen.

Want to take out your toxic trash, nourish your organs, prevent cancer, and keep Baby's metaphorical fridge stocked with nutrients? Go take a walk in nature. Thanks to the flowers and the trees and the birds and the bees, there is more oxygen where the breeze blows.

Stress Relief

The goal of all stress-relieving activities is to get you to breathe more deeply. Relaxation recording? You end up breathing deeper. Exercise? You have no choice but to suck in more oxygen. The more you practice taking deep breaths the moment something stressful occurs, the easier it will be for you to reach your Meditation Room without spending much time in the Panic Room.

Clarity of Thought

"Pregnancy brain" thrives when we're not breathing. On a particularly stressful day of my pregnancy I slathered ghee (clarified butter) on my face instead of sunscreen, forgot to wear panties under a white muumuu, and drove to the grocery store without shoes. The struggle is real.

If you'll need to continue functioning in society during pregnancy, you'll need a few doses of clarity of thought. Whenever you find yourself struggling to grasp a coherent thought, or to remember why you walked into your closet, *stop*, close your eyes, and take five *deep* inhalations and *slow* exhalations.

Oxygen Makes You Happy

When you're taking full breaths, your pleasure-inducing alpha brain waves are stimulated, which promotes the release of beta-endorphins. Focused breathing also tells your overstimulated neurotransmitters that it's time to chill. While oxygen is making you physically happy, it also gives your spirit and emotions a little tickle, reminding them to cheer up. Deep breathing is one of the rare acts that unify your mind, body, and spirit in one fell swoop.

Muscle Maintenance

Oxygen is the lifeblood of your muscles. Without oxygen, your muscles would not have the energy to do what they need to do, especially during birth.

You breathe more when you exercise. Why? Your muscles are telling you that they need more fuel to accomplish the tasks you're asking them to perform. You breathe more when you give birth. Why? Your muscles are telling you that they need more fuel to accomplish the task you're asking them to perform.

When your muscles are not receiving enough oxygen but are still being pushed, they stop creating energy, and start to convert glucose into lactic acid, causing *an*-aerobic exercise. Translated from Greek, *anaerobic* means "living without air." Anaerobic exercise quickly leads to fatigue; if the physical activity you happen to be partaking in is birth, fatigue could open the door to interventions. That list of birth preferences you're creating? Continuous deep breathing during birth (even if it initially feels like one of the hardest acts you've ever said yes to) will help you bring many of those preferences to fruition.

Breathing Makes You Svelte

Deep belly breathing helps you burn more calories. This is the kind of breathing that causes the lower belly to be pushed out. Ironically, one of the reasons deep belly breathing feels so unnatural to many is because our culture values (a.k.a. "is obsessed with") flat bellies, and we avoid anything that gives the belly extra "pooch," even for an instant. Lucky for you, you're pregnant, and the pooch is smiled upon. Take this time of "pooch acceptance" as an opportunity to train your body to fill all areas of your lungs (not just the top part) with oxygen.

Here's how allowing your lower belly to move with each breath helps you burn off fat:

1. Your body needs energy to function. Even when you're sleeping, your body is using energy. Where does this energy come from? Glycogen.

2. Glycogen is a form of sugar your body uses to create ATP (adenosine triphosphate), the high-energy molecule that stores the energy you need to do just about everything — this is what your body runs on.

3. Oxygen converts food into glucose, which creates the store of gly-cogen. The less oxygen surging through you, the less glycogen being converted into energy, and the less fat being burned.

4. Without a healthy supply of oxygen, your stubborn stores of fat cannot be sizzled off.

To sum it up, oxygen speeds up the metabolism and helps you burn off the additional piece of pie you ate after your partner went to bed.

Breathing Improves Your Posture

Hunch over and try to take a deep breath. Now, stand up straight and try to take a deep breath. Which breath felt more effective?

Being conscious of your breath and training your mind to take more enriching breaths will help you become more aware of your body. When you're aware of your body, hunching over will just seem wrong. The Breath-Hampering Hunch causes the muscles of your chest to constrict, prevents the rib cage from properly expanding, stresses your already pissed-off back muscles, stagnates the life force of energy running through your spine, con-stricts your baby's range of motion, and causes your organs, specifically the ones supporting Baby's growth and protection, to work harder. You don't deserve all that noise. Breathe deeply on the regular, and your body will naturally align, giving all your bits and pieces the room, and the correct positioning, to function without complaint.

If you feel the urge to forgo proper posture to ease weariness, go lie down on your side, stick a pillow between your legs, and take a nap. If you're stuck up the creek without a paddle (e.g., stuck in traffic with a full bladder and heavy lids), force yourself to sit up straight, or pull over if you're in dan-ger of falling asleep. Did you know good posture also helps to ease the agony of a full bladder and increases your energy?

Good posture begets good posture. If you've become accustomed to the slouch, it may feel like a cruel exercise in futility to stand or sit up straight, but the more you practice good posture, in conjunction with deep breathing, the more natural it will become. (And erect posture also makes you appear slimmer. Cheers to optical illusions!)

How to Release Your Uterus from the Fear-Tension-Pain Syndrome

When you are fearful, you experience tension; when you are tense, you experience pain; and when you experience pain, more fear is birthed — and round and round you go.

How the heck do you get out of this energy-sucking cycle? One of the most integral tools for saving yourself from fear-tension-pain (FTP) hysteria is to breathe deeply. This is easier when the challenge you're experiencing is primarily mental because your body has more disposable attention to focus on breath work and support you in settling the mind and emotions. It gets trickier when your body is distracted by childbirth.

During birth, you will experience surges. These surges are your body's natural means for birthing your baby. As a surge begins, the outer, vertical muscles of your uterus will pull up and out, then gently give Baby a nudge down. As these vertical muscles pull up, out, and down, they open and unfold the inner, circular muscles of your uterus, which are most concentrated near your cervix. That's it, that's how your body births your baby. So simple, right? Then why is birth so difficult for so many women?

Many women do not breathe properly during birth and swirl in the FTP cycle the entire time, making birth very unpleasant. When the uterus (not to mention the baby) is not provided with enough space and oxygen to do its birthing dance unencumbered, pain occurs. This pain occurs when a woman holds her breath, or takes shallow breaths, causing her muscles to contract. It's not easy moving a baby through contracted muscles. Because it's unlikely your vertical uterine muscles will cease surging once labor has begun (and you don't want them to take too long of a break if you're hoping for a vaginal birth), your circular uterine muscles will continue to be pulled upward, no matter how taut they are. When taut muscles are forcefully pulled, serious discomfort occurs. When those circular muscles are made loose and pliable by deep breath work, they cooperate and open without much fuss.

You don't have to drown in the FTP cycle. Practice the following breathing techniques *every day*, so your body organically supports your birthing efforts.

De-stressor Breathing

This is the breath work you'll utilize now to soothe common stressors, and in between surges during birth. When you've practiced this enough, you may notice yourself always breathing to this pattern (and people commenting on how incessantly calm you are).

Do this:

1. Inhale to a slow count of eight.
2. Hold for three.
3. Release to a slow count of eight.
4. Continue until you're settled in your mental Meditation Room.

Labor Breathing (during Surges)

Use this breath through each surge; you'll likely need to do a few during each surge. This breath creates extra room and oxygen for your baby, reducing your chances of needing interventions, and prevents the tension between your outer and inner uterine muscles.

Do this:

1. Slowly inhale to a quick count from one to as high as you can count.
2. Slowly exhale to the same count.

The numbers don't matter as much as the intention behind the breath does. If you can only reach ten or eleven when you first start practicing, that's fine. Take pride as your numbers grow each time you practice.

Use one of the following visualizations with each Labor Breath:

- Pretend a rose is unfolding with each inhalation and closing with each exhalation.
- Imagine the oxygen being sent to your baby and uterus is a bright light infused with love and pain relief.
- Envision your body turning into warm, pliable goo with each exhalation.

Descent Breathing

After you have moved through transition, have come to feel a strong fullness in your rectum and pelvis, and you're fully dilated (at 10 cm), you may not sense an urge to bear down. If you don't feel an overwhelming compulsion to push and you're still experiencing surges (sometimes surges take a brief pause after transition), practice this Descent Breathing, which you can also use in conjunction with pushing.

Use this breathing only during surges; in between surges use the De-stressor Breath to conserve your energy.

Do this:

1. Do a quick and strong inhalation.
2. Envision your exhalation being pushed down the back of your throat, through the uterus, and out your vaginal opening, and en-vision your baby being nudged down and out. This breath sounds similar to the Ujjayi yoga breath.
3. Repeat.

If your body tells you it's ready to bear down, do this breathing as you push down. This breath stimulates your natural expulsive reflex, the same reflex your body uses to push waste out of your intestines. So it feels just like you're having a bowel movement, but instead of poop you'll get a baby! You can practice this breath during bowel movements.

Perineal Tissue Massage

You'll be more confident moving into birth if you've already experienced the power your breath has to minimize discomfort, specifically in your perineal region, the opening your baby will come out of. Perineal tissue massage is less of a massage and more of a "vagina stretching" — helping the skin and muscles that make up your perineum become more pliable and willing to create space for a big baby head. This is one of the best (physical) actions you can take to prepare for birth, as you'll notice increased suppleness in your vaginal opening each time you do it, and your mind will become more of a champ at learning to chill the F out as you move through an uncomfortable experience.

Move through the following routine daily, beginning six weeks before your Guess Due Time.

Do this:

1. Put a few tablespoons of a single-ingredient oil (e.g., coconut or jojoba oil) into a shallow cup or bowl.

2. Take off your undies and go somewhere private. The toilet may be the easiest location for this, as it provides ample access to your vagina. If your partner is up for the get-down (or the get-in), ask them to do this for you.

3. Turn on your favorite relaxation recording, take some De-stressor or Labor Breaths, and envision your perineum unfolding like a flower, or a fleshy kaleidoscope. (Like that visual?)

4. Set a timer for five to ten minutes.

5. Next, dip your thumb, or your pointer and middle finger, in your shallow oil dish.

6. Insert the thumb or fingers about two inches into your vaginal opening and move them in a horseshoe-like motion down toward your rectum and back up again, keeping your fingers inserted at the same depth the entire time. Continue this back and forth motion.

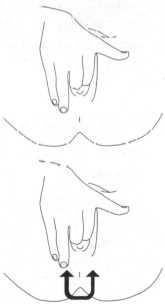

7. Start gently to find your rhythm, then progressively begin to widen "the horseshoe" so you begin to feel more pressure and stretching in your perineum. If you feel discomfort, practice De-Stressor or Labor Breathing through it.

8. When the timer goes off, rub the residual oil into your vagina and wash off your hands.

9. Pat yourself on the tush and honor yourself for putting in the effort to create a well-prepared perineum. A stretchy perineum is a happy perineum.

From Her Heart to Yours

I've always been a chronic breath-holder. The phrase "just breathe" has always bothered me — "I can't *just breathe!* I don't know how!" Pregnancy forced me to learn how. I experienced a wicked version of "the sickness" every trimester of pregnancy — my tooth-brushing endeavors often ended with me heaving bile into the toilet. During my childbirth preparation course (which I unfortunately did not take until the middle of my third trimester), I learned three breathing techniques: two helped me stop vomiting and the third helped me stop getting constipated. It's like the breaths were the "lovey" for my tummy. And labor? I initially envisioned myself puking through each surge — instead, I breathed through each surge and didn't regurgitate a single ice chip! Now when I see someone struggling with their pregnancy, I tell them to *just breathe* — and yes, the advice is usually unsolicited.

— *R. T., San Antonio, Texas (mom to three boys who love to talk about vomit and other bodily functions)*

RIDDLE: Hi! I'm the type of breath that helps you poop. What's my name?

Go to **YourSereneLife.wordpress.com/chapter-seventeen** and use the two-word riddle answer as your offer code to download the relaxation recording for this chapter!

CALL TO PLEASURE

❧❧❧

- Practice De-Stressor Breathing daily: inhale for eight, hold for three, then exhale for eight.
- Practice Labor Breathing when waking up and going to bed: slow inhale to a quick count from one to as high as you can go, then slow exhale to the same count.

- Practice Descent Breathing during bowel movements: strong inhale, then powerful exhale directed down the back of the throat, through the uterus, and out the vaginal opening.
- Practice De-Stressor or Labor Breathing while doing a five-to-ten-minute perineal tissue massage, daily, beginning six weeks before your Guess Due Time.

CHAPTER EIGHTEEN

ENHANCING SPIRITUAL HEALTH:
Caressing Your Sacral Chakra

JUST BREATHE: *As you inhale, allow the oxygen to awaken each of the seven chakras as it flows through you, touching first on the chakra at the base of your spine, then second on the chakra in your navel, next the chakra in the pit of your stomach, moving into the chakra in your heart, flowing into the chakra in your throat, waking up the chakra in your third eye, and finally arousing the chakra in the crown of your head.*

Your sacral chakra, located in your lower abdomen, is the home of your baby's soul, and it is supporting the growth of a new chakra system. The growth of this new system throws your own system out of whack; it needs help pulling itself back into alignment. It's crucial to dissolve any blocks in your sacral chakra before you move into birth, as these blocks could dampen your ability to bond with Baby. Releasing these blocks through rituals woven into this chapter will awaken your birthright of fully connecting with your Baby Love.

What the Heck Is the Chakra System?

Your body has seven chakras, or energy centers, believed to be your spiritual hotbeds. But they're not always happy hotbeds — sometimes they're just hot*heads* that need some soothing and unclogging. The chakras begin with the first chakra at the base of your spine and are oriented all the way to the seventh chakra at the top of your head. Each chakra is aligned with a certain area of your body, and with specific emotions.

- **First chakra (red):** This is your root chakra, composed of the energy housed in the base of your spine. This is where your primal survival instincts, groundedness, and trust in your intuition hang out. When this chakra is happy, you move into birth with deep trust for your body, your baby, your supporters, and your ability to make empowered decisions. Give a hug to this chakra by spending time with your feet in the earth, feeling yourself becoming heavier and heavier the longer you stand, as if your body is sinking down into the ground.

- **Second chakra (orange):** Your sacral chakra is located in your pelvic region, a crucial area in the whole baby-birthing thing. We'll burrow deep into this chakra in this chapter.

- **Third chakra (yellow):** This energy center, located in your solar plexus (the pit of your stomach), fosters confidence, composure, and the warrior woman within. This assuredness helps you move into the unknown of childbirth and motherhood with a knowing you will hold the power to follow through on your convictions and the pursuit of your desires. For example, your third chakra is in balance when you stand up for your birth preferences and cosleeping even though your mother-in-law's eyebrow twitches every time you mention it. Learn to honor the signals of this chakra by closing your eyes, placing your hands slightly above your belly button, and asking the question you need an answer to (e.g., "Should I accept the synthetic oxytocin being offered?"). If you feel churning, nausea, or another form of discomfort in your solar plexus, this could be your intuition giving you a "no," and if you feel a lightening, warmth, or other comfortable sensation, that could be a "yes." Practice this technique with smaller dilemmas before you go into labor, to develop a trust for the messages offered by this chakra.

- **Fourth chakra (green):** This is your heart chakra, the source of compassion, generosity, and your ability to offer and receive love. When this warm center is in balance, bonding with Baby (even before birth) is easier, and those annoying habits your partner has won't bother you as much. To nurture this chakra, place your hands over your heart and repeat the mantra, "I am an infinite source of love." You can offer the same mantra to your baby when he is born.

- **Fifth chakra (blue):** This is the chakra living within and around your throat, and it's crucial to your ability to communicate. This chakra not only is important for verbal communication; it also allows your intuition to speak through your breathing, facial expressions, and posture, all of which are especially important during birth, when you may need to express your needs without actually having to talk. To open that voice, slowly sip water or a warm beverage (free of caffeine), envisioning any lumps or other barriers being flushed out of your throat.

- **Sixth chakra (indigo):** Did you know you have a third eye, right in the middle of your forehead? Yup. And that's right where this indigo chakra has planted itself. When the energy in this knowing "eye" is balanced, you trust your inner wisdom to guide and support you. If you're having trouble making decisions (especially during the emotionally charged moments of birth), close your eyes and look up toward the middle of your forehead, begin emitting a low hum to clear your mind, and allow the voice of your intuition to speak to you.

- **Seventh chakra (purple):** The energy in the crown of your head floats partially in you and partially in the spirit realm (if you subscribe to energy from that realm). If you feel yourself lacking a connection to "something more," to an "all-encompassing source of love," tune in to the sensations in the top of your head, envisioning a warm light spreading over it and enlivening the energy in that space.

Because these chakras do not exist in bubbles, each one interacts with and affects the others; it's favorable to give them all TLC on the regular by following the suggestions offered. But, because the sacral chakra is equal parts vulnerable and crucial during the mega-expedition you're on, we're going to give it a few more spa treatments (metaphorical or literal — the sacral chakra is so down for a mud bath and massage).

Why You Should Care about Your Sacral Chakra

The sacral chakra, your mind-body-spirit superglue, is known as the "dwelling place of the Self" and promotes a whole-being cohesiveness. When your glue comes apart, fear, sexual disinterest, and melancholy sneak in. When it's feeling good, this chakra promotes well-being, joy, gratification, and abundance and is always on the hunt for pleasure, passion, sensuality, and connection. This energy center will also help you feel sexy in your transitioning body and accept your plumping with love, or at least good-natured tolerance.

Brewing good juju in your sacral chakra will help you *feel into* the sensations of birth, giving you more power to steer them in the direction you like (probably a less uncomfortable direction). When you're birthing from a space where you're filled with and surrounded by vibrant energy in your baby-birthing zone, you're able to release, move into, and honor the shifts of childbirth, placing you fully in the experience of each moment. When you access this sweet spot of "in the moment—

P.S. *The sacral chakra also has a strong connection to your lower back, which often takes the brunt of labor sensations.*

ness" during childbirth, you no longer care how long your birth is; all you need to do is move through one moment at a time.

In addition to the sacral chakra acting as glue for your mind-body-spirit, it also serves as an alert system for it, doing periodic sweeps for lingering junk to support the fear-release work you've begun. These sweeps and junk alerts come in the form of uncomfortable sensations in your lower abdomen, serving as a signal that you need to free trapped negativity by going back to your fear-release work (e.g., a ninety-second exercise, journaling, fear-release meditation, deep breathing, etc.).

Your Sacral Chakra Needs to Poop

Why is this chakra often the most constipated one? In most individuals the full expression of this chakra is suppressed in early childhood, when our culture teaches us to stifle our emotions in favor of putting up a happy front to make those around us more comfortable. The barricades around this energy center are frequently fortified in adulthood because the fire of our creative expression has wet towels continually thrown on it from the time we leave elementary school. "Do what you're supposed to you. Follow along with the rest of us. Don't be weird."

The sacral chakra loves it when social norms are thrown out and you conjure up some original ideas. And because it's pleased when we become comfortable with failure, or with situations not turning the way we originally wanted them to turn, it's confused by the constant avoidance of failure and the obsession with control many cultures promote. Making your sacral chakra happy by releasing these futile needs will send you into childbirth open and willing to accept the unpredictable nature of the experience. Hey, Girl, belly dance in the dairy aisle of the grocery store to release that bellyache — who gives a hoot if people look at you funny? (They're probably constipated.)

How to Spill Love on Your Sacral Chakra

All of the bullet points in this section are juicy kisses for your sacral chakra, but there is no need for a make-out session; doing them all would create too much spiritual saliva. Read through all the suggestions, tune in to those that create a warmth and lightness in your lower abdomen, and then regularly practice those.

- **Creation:** Garden, find solutions to a challenge, write, draw, turn something raw and unfinished into something beautiful, make something where there was nothing. (Building a baby = ultimate creation?)
- **Release attachment:** This includes releasing your attachment to the finished product of the actions you take; make it all about the process instead. For example, when you're cooking, don't just yearn to have the finished food in your mouth; savor the aroma of the cilantro while you're chopping, the crispness of the celery as you slice it, or the satisfaction of smashing the heck out of those cooked potatoes.
- **Invent something!** A new recipe. A solution to global warming. Whatever.
- **Go play!**
- **Have sex!**
- **Pelvic gyrations:** Want to kill two birds with one pelvis? Do pelvic swirls while engaging in the previous suggestion. Emotional and physical tension tends to gather in your hips and pelvic region, and you'll need more than happy thoughts to release it.

- **Dance:** Dance like your hippie friends are watching. Dance to the rhythm of some music, dance to your own rhythm, make strange sounds while you move. Get freaky with it!
- **Strengthen your core:** Strong abdominal muscles create a safe and happy home for your sacral chakra. On the daily, practice yoga, swim, or walk, all while pulling your abdominal muscles in and up (as much as is comfortable for you; don't suck in your belly and hold your breath — we don't want to suffocate our chakras).
- **Meditate on sending orange light to your sacral chakra** — it looks best in that color. This tangy visualization promotes enhanced cellular health, more gentle handling of your emotions, and a long life.
- **Walk on the Earth:** *Feel* the Earth.

Sacral Chakra Affirmations

Pick one or two of these daily. Close your eyes, place your hands over your lower abdomen, and repeat your selected affirmations one at a time, envisioning the message being absorbed by your "mama chakra."

- I love my body unconditionally.
- I soak in the current moment with all my senses.
- I liberate my latent feelings and emotions.
- I savor my sexuality.
- I give life to my primal desires by breathing into them, instead of suppressing them.
- I am open to loving touch.
- I nurture my body with the food and drink that I'm intuitively drawn to.
- I accept pleasure.
- I release guilt.

From My Heart to Yours

Chakra talk in yoga used to piss me off because I had no idea what they were talking about. "Feel into your third chakra." What the heck? But when I learned "Chakras for Dummies" in my childbirth preparation training, I was converted. I didn't dive into the intricate profiles of each chakra, but I got the gist, learning how to "feel into" them and give 'em some love. When I started a morning meditation of scanning each of my chakras, I noticed that I always felt soreness in the center of my forehead, my sixth chakra. I realized I was completely disconnected from my intuition, always listening to what others thought was best, not what I felt to be best. I began ending my meditations with an intuition-awakening exercise, asking myself different questions and listening to the first answer that came up, via the voice of my intuition. A week after doing this the soreness in my forehead was gone.

— *Bailey Gaddis, Ojai, California (chakra enthusiast)*

RIDDLE: I'm the chakra that's the color of the ocean — where do I live?

Go to **YourSereneLife.wordpress.com/chapter-eighteen** and use the one-word riddle answer as your offer code to download the relaxation recording for this chapter!

CALL TO PLEASURE

- Choose a sampling of your favorite chakra-loving activities and #JustDoIt.
- Daily, eat one of the foods or flavors the sacral chakra craves (e.g., orange, mango, vanilla, or almond).
- Each time you feel hormonal upheaval, find a private space and meditate on what area of your chakra feels most affected. For example, if your throat feels tight, your fifth chakra is being constrained. Then, do the activity or activities mentioned to clear that chakra.

FOURTH TRIMESTER

FIRST STEPS
into
NEW LIFE

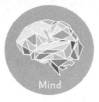
Mind

CHAPTER NINETEEN

MAINTAINING SOME "ME" TIME

JUST BREATHE! *As you practice this breathing exercise, allow a deep awareness of your authentic Self, whatever you sense that to be, to begin waking up. Now, breathe in to a slow count of ten, focusing on sending all the energy of the breath into your heart center. As you breathe out, allow latent guilt to flow out of your heart center.*

Without daily doses of self-love, your coffer of New Mama Special Sauce will run dry. You need time to nourish your body, your passions, your creativity, and your spirituality to keep up this whole coherence thing people keep saying is important. Steel yourself now to push through the icy wall of resistance that stands between your Guilty Self and the Self that feels okay taking time away from your baby to pull yourself back together. This may be the chapter you're tempted to skim through or even (gasp!) skip, to get to the "important" stuff, the righteous stuff that equally focuses on your baby's needs — because that's all you have time for, right? *Wrong.* If you don't throw yourself a bone every day, your reserves will run dry quicker than a leaky boob soaks through a thin shirt. So read this chapter! Your whole being is so worthy of doting.

This chapter will teach you how to self-dote by setting aside time and space for your needs, even when your heart (and likely a chunk of your brain) is hanging with your new baby. You'll learn practical techniques to build your self-care muscles so that in the ecstatic chaos of new motherhood, you don't lose your ability to care for yourself. And because your former identity did not die when you birthed your baby (it just had a spiritual face-lift), we'll focus on honoring the twin blossoms of your dual identity as an individual and as someone's mother.

You Can Still Be You

Public Service Announcement: You don't need to trade in your prebaby identity for a minivan. Your sense of Self is not deposited behind your placenta. Your partner will still be really interested in getting it on with you. You are now a mom, but you're still a woman.

While you are committing to waking up every few hours for feedings and keeping the poop situation under control, please don't neglect to commit to a bit of autonomy. Because Girl, if the woman inside the mama doesn't get regular turns to come out and play, she may lash out.

Honoring your right to still be *you* will also make you a better mother. Your baby didn't choose the burp rag–slinging, stretchy pants–wearing, vaccine research–obsessed you (as fun as these new aspects of your Self are) — she chose the woman who honored her own needs, passions, creative inclinations, and spiritual cravings. You don't need to assume a new identity to be a good mother. Your new role as mother will organically mold you over time into the best version of yourself, so the pressure is off. No need to force yourself into mommy-approved classes you're not drawn to, ways of speaking that make you think "who is this person?" — or other ways of being and doing that don't feel authentic. Your growing love for your baby will support you in blossoming into the unique version of Mother you need to be for the child who chose *you.*

Oh, wait; have the insane concoctions of hormones mixed with stroller research made you forget who the heck you are? Here's an exercise to help you reintegrate with that rad lady at your core:

1. Describe your Self (before you became pregnant) in three words. Now, describe that Self in one paragraph.
2. Write out the traits, skills, friends, dreams, beauty products, sex positions, foods, *whatever* that you dug about your pre-pregnancy life, things you'd like to integrate into your current life.

3. Then, list all the aspects of that past life you'd like to shed during this mommy metamorphosis.

4. Now, do free-flow writing, examining everything: all the things you miss, what you're excited about, the aspects of yourself you're confused about, the mind-blowing experience of staring at your new human, how your romantic relationship has shifted…let it flow.

5. Finally, set a timer for ten minutes, close your eyes, and sit with how you feel after scribbling your Self onto paper.

How to Connect with You

Now that you've been reintroduced to your core Self, you should wine and dine her — or just take her to bed. *Knowing* that your unique Self is in there is not enough; she needs regular acknowledgment and nurturing to stake her claim in your new life. Many of the women I've worked with who had postpartum blues described feeling like a shell, absorbed by the title of "Mom," unable to connect with what brought them joy, or sad they didn't find happiness in the activities that moms "should find happiness in." It was as though their true Self had been snipped along with the umbilical cord, and they were relying on motherhood to connect them to a sense of fulfillment and purpose. That's way too much pressure on your baby, and on motherhood. Sure, those are both big, honking components in your life, but they're not everything.

Use these activities to revive your dedication to your core (sexy-creative-passionate-capable-adventurous) Self:

•   **Discover your bare minimum of alone time.** We all place different orders for alone time. Some people need ample solitary time — no one touching them, talking to them, or giving them sidelong glances, none of that. Others thrive on connection and can refill their solo-tank in a matter of minutes. Where do you lie on this spectrum?

    Over the next few days, experiment with your timing — one day asking your partner to keep the baby for thirty minutes while you do what you please, the next day requesting an hour, or one thirty-minute chunk in the morning and one in the evening. Play around with time. At the end of each day, sink into how you feel, noticing whether you feel satisfied with the amount of self-imposed solitary confinement you received. Once you settle on your sweet spot, advocate for receiving this amount of alone time each day. Schedule it in.

- **Meditate:** There is just as much accomplishment in meditation as there is in answering your emails, folding laundry, or finally finishing the lotus flower in your adult coloring book. Set your timer (for ten, twenty, forty-five minutes?), close your eyes, and just sit. Things curiously begin to fall into place when meditation is a part of your daily diet.

- **Take a nap (alone):** I place sleep on the same pedestal as meditation. Closing your eyes and lying on a comfortable surface is not a luxury, it's a requirement. If your alone time comes around and you feel pressure behind your eyes, an ache in your body, and a desire to scream into a pillow, you probably need some sleep. You'll be better at life after you get some sleep. And the excuse "I'll just sleep when the baby sleeps" doesn't fly. You sleep differently, and better, alone, when your baby is in someone else's care, because then you can fully release and settle into that deeply efficient slumber where your body can turn into mush.

- **Mix prescheduled activities with spontaneity:** It's easy to spend half of your alone time figuring out what you want to do with your alone time. Preschedule about two-thirds of your alone time (for example, have a set activity planned for your Monday, Wednesday, Thursday, and Saturday alone time), and leave the other third open to spontaneity. For the planned days, select activities you know will make your soul buzz, like meditating then writing, or going for a walk and calling your best friend. Then, when you have a spontaneous day, sit in a moment of silence and ask yourself, "What do I feel like doing right now?" Then, honor the answer.

- **Respect your bliss!** For the love of sleeping babies, honor what brings you bliss. I guarantee that ticking off boxes on your to-do list does not compare to serving your mind-body-spirit what it truly craves. These cravings commonly take the form of creative tinkerings, activities that make you sweat, or the aforementioned meditation or sleep. Do what makes you feel good and forget the rest, knowing the rest will eventually get done.

How to Show the Love to Your Partner

Remember that person who supported you in the baby-conjuring process? They were likely a big kahuna in your prebaby life, which makes them an anchor for your prebaby Self. Your connection to your partner should not be an afterthought; keeping the love cycling between the two of you will allow the love to continue pouring into Baby. As lovely as babies are, they demand much more than they can give; in moments when all you need is a hug and kiss, the baby may just give you a fat wail and epic spit-up down your boobs. Babies are not in the position to give you what you need when you need it, but your partner is, at least most of the time.

When you're too tired to remember how to show the love to the other adult in your house, utilize the following suggestions:

- **Just do it:** When you feel ready, just *do* the sex. I know you're tired, I know they're tired — but how often have you moved through all the moves and regretted it, especially if the moves end in orgasm? And heck, if you both fall asleep halfway through, you needed it.
- **Make eye contact:** Connecting to your partner does not always need to include physical touch; sitting in front of each other and noticing the intricacies of one another's eyes can be deeply intimate (and maybe awkward at first, but just go with it). If you choose to talk during your time together, ensure you're staying committed to the conversation by looking into the cosmos of your honey's peepers.
- **Be here now:** Avoid talking about scheduling, or diaper brands, or college savings plans during your baby-less time. Settle into The Now by talking about the feelings in your body in this moment, or the random thoughts popping up — just see where it leads you. Let the goal be to let out silly or romantic expression, not productivity. You can compare the merits of Montessori and Waldorf preschools another day.
- **Remember why you fell in love:** If you move into your time with your partner feeling frustrated about something they have, or have

not, been doing, spend some time thinking about and *sharing with them* all their "ways of being" that first made you fall in love with them. Then, if you still feel like you need to express your frustrations you'll move into the conversation in a more loving manner, and they'll be less likely to be defensive. You are together for a reason; let the love that lives in that reason be your guiding light.

Scheduling

Ugh, scheduling — boring! But important it is, Mama Grasshopper. Getting down with the art of scheduling frees your mind-body-spirit amalgam to spend its time dancing in the space of enjoyment and exploration, rather than trying to remember if it's supposed to be at your mother-in-law's house or the metal stirrups in your OB's office at 2:00 PM. Use the following strategies to sync up with the magic of writing that stuff down, and honoring the written word of your schedule.

- **Find your apparatus of choice:** Phone app, notebook, dry-erase board, Etch-a-Sketch, day timer — if you can write words on it, you can use it to record your schedule. Find a schedule device that suits your needs, and use it! I recommend a portable device you can stash in your purse or diaper bag, so you can jot down a thought or to-do the moment it pops up. Have only *one* place where you record your schedule; the confusion of having more than one planning device is mental torture.
- **Record everything immediately:** The scheduling device is a worthless piece of extra stuff if you don't transform it into an Essential with your words. Write words in that planner, right when you think of the words.
- **Put your appointments and essential to-dos in the same place:** Kiss your mind by keeping all that important stuff in the same place. Beginning your passion project is just as important as your dentist appointment, so put them both on the same schedule. And remember, your "me time" counts as an essential to-do that deserves a spot on your schedule.

- **Schedule flexibility:** Ironically, scheduling the essential activities of your day leaves more room for flexibility. When you fail to schedule the essential activities, what often happens is your "flexible time" is siphoned away by trying to remember what you're supposed to be doing. So don't fill in every gap of your daily schedule with stuff; leave big gaps where you and Baby can do what you feel like doing, allowing your day to breathe instead of being strangled by constant obligations.

- **Stick to the schedule (and sometimes don't):** Respect thy schedule. It may take a while for you to get used to ending an activity at a set time, in favor of beginning something else that is important to you. But as you deepen your groove in the process of schedule-making-and-honoring, you'll end your days drenched in a really lovely state of accomplishment and fulfilled purpose. (And then, there will be days when all hell breaks loose and you need to let your schedule take a nap.)

From My Heart to Yours

#GuiltyMommyConfession: When my son was a newborn I committed more energy to scheduling my solo-time activities than his sleep and feeding schedules. I tried the reverse for a while and no one was happy; I became so obsessed with ensuring he kept his eyes closed at the "appropriate" times and accepted my leaky boobs only when my timer went off that there was no energy left to figure out nurturing ways to spend time with myself. When I tinkered with scrapping the baby schedule in favor of scheduling my own nurturing, Hudson and I settled. Because I was using *my* time emerged in activities that lit my fire, I returned to my son calm, playful, and more receptive to his ever-shifting needs. The times he ate and slept slightly varied every day, but it organically fell into a pattern that best suited his needs.

— *Bailey Gaddis, Ojai, California*

RIDDLE: What "sitting up straight, eyes closed, timer set" activity should you engage in daily? Even if it's just for three minutes?

Go to **YourSereneLife.wordpress.com/chapter-nineteen** and use the one-word riddle answer as your offer code to download the relaxation recording for this chapter.

CALL TO PLEASURE

- Determine what your bare minimum amount of alone time is each day and commit to claiming that period for yourself. Set up a schedule with your partner or other trusted loved one, so they can care for Baby during that time. Just do it.
- Preschedule about two-thirds of your alone time. Your time is made of precious drops of moments that you don't want to waste on rumination over what to do.
- Set aside regular periods of time where you connect with your partner: have sex, talk about anything but your baby, make eye contact, cuddle and nap, do whatever makes you feel more connected to your love muffin.
- Select a scheduling apparatus of choice and use that sucker. Write down all your appointments and essential to-dos, then *follow your schedule.*

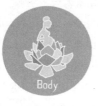

CHAPTER TWENTY

BREASTFEEDING:
Dissolving the Mystery of the Liquid Gold

JUST BREATHE: *As you inhale, envision your milk ducts expanding, and as you exhale, envision them filling with milk. Then go feed that baby (if he's out of the womb).*

Offer the breast and forget the rest. Seriously, if you scrap most of the baby stuff, sleep advice, swaddle strategies, and other useful-but-not-essential baby items and ideas and just breastfeed (a lot), you and Baby will be golden. If it's physically possible for you, breastfeeding is the best way to nurture the emotional and physical health of your baby. Breastfeeding has been found to lower the risk of childhood leukemia, increase IQ, and promote mother-baby bonding, and it boasts a catalog of impressive additional benefits. Breastfeeding is the tits.

This chapter reveals the bounty of goodness breastfeeding holds for you and your baby, and I hope it will boost your confidence and resolve to choose this method of nourishing, if possible. In this chapter, I will discuss breastfeeding positions, latch techniques, timing considerations, the amount of milk you can expect to produce, and additional information that will demystify this natural — but not always easy — form of feeding. This is an area of new motherhood where so many of us are undersupported and isolated. It is my goal to clarify breastfeeding and offer support to you, especially if you're finding nursing successfully to be challenging. (I'll also teach you how to avoid waking up in a warm pond of sticky breast milk.)

Please note that you can still "nurse" even when you're bottle-feeding. For various reasons, some parents are not able to breastfeed, and that in no way means your baby is any less likely to win Olympic Gold, crest the summit of Everest, or write the next Earth-shattering novel. Simply setting aside sacred time to feed and connect with your baby will accomplish emotional benefits synonymous with those breastfeeding mamas and babies enjoy. Bottle-feeding your baby can even cause a release of oxytocin within you, without any nipple stimulation needed!

Health Benefits for Baby

A study done by the National Institute of Environmental Health Sciences showed that children who are breastfed have a 20 percent lower risk of dying between the ages of twenty-eight days and one year than children who weren't breastfed. In addition, a large German study published in 2009 found that breastfeeding — either exclusively or partially — is associated with a lower risk of sudden infant death syndrome (SIDS). The researchers concluded that exclusive breastfeeding at one month of age cut the risk of SIDS in half. The U.S. Centers for Disease Control and Prevention (CDC) recommends breastfeeding for as long as possible to reduce the risk of SIDS. Boom. Mic drop.

Want some more? Breastfeeding lowers your child's chance of contracting childhood leukemia, stomach viruses, lower respiratory illnesses, ear infections, and meningitis and decreases her chances of developing allergies or becoming obese.

But breast milk isn't just interested in keeping the physical functions of the body on point; it's also been suggested that breastfeeding improves cognitive development. A study published in the journal *JAMA Pediatrics* found that children received higher test scores the longer they were breastfed. In addition, breastfeeding can save your baby in the case of an emergency: it requires no water, protecting her from the effects of a contaminated water supply; it keeps you snuggled, helping to prevent hypothermia; and it requires zero supplies.

So how does breastfeeding create all these organic miracles? Continuing research is suggesting that your milk is custom made for your baby, with your milk ducts containing sensors that pick up signals in your baby's saliva that tell your body what your baby's unique body requires. Your body then responds by creating custom milk! Your tatas also serve up a regular helping of vitamins, nutrients, and other disease-fighting substances, serving as natural immunizations for your baby the first few months of her life. Your body does this by responding to pathogens you're exposed to and producing custom milk that helps protect your baby from the pathogens' potential harmful effects.

The crown jewel of this super-powered milk is colostrum, or your "first milk." Colostrum, a yellowish milk you will secrete for the first one or two days of your baby's life, includes a substance that wards off germs by creating a protective layer over mucous membranes in Baby's intestines, nose, and throat. This golden goodness is also full of carbohydrates, proteins, and antibodies, which give Baby an extra boost of healthy and protect her from multiple bacteria and viruses right from the start. Colostrum also has a laxative effect, helping excess bilirubin (the culprit behind jaundice) and that tar oil–like meconium poop make their way down and out of Baby. Among people who have not been properly educated on breastfeeding, new mothers who see this yellow milk might believe their milk is bad and stop breastfeeding in favor of formula. Spread your knowledge.

For these reasons, both the American Academy of Pediatrics and the World Health Organization recommend exclusive breastfeeding for the first six months of Baby's life. The American Academy of Pediatrics recommends continuing to breastfeed, in addition to offering safe supplemental food, at least until your baby is one, while the World Health Organization recommends breastfeeding, in addition to food, for at least two years.

Health Benefits for You

Breastfeeding is not only kind to Baby, it can be the one act that gives you reprieve from many of the arduous surprises (like lingering weight, deep moments of funk, or an unexpected positive pregnancy test) you may encounter in the months after the cord has been cut.

Here are the specific benefits your mind and body can expect when you breastfeed:

- Helps the uterus contract and reduces chance of excessive postpartum bleeding.
- Provides an exit from the postpartum emotional roller coaster, and a potential barrier to postpartum depression. The natural feel-good hormone oxytocin is released when you nurse, promoting relaxation and soothing your nerves. The release of oxytocin may also cause a flood of sleepiness; if you're in a comfortable location, give in to the calm and take an oxytocin-enhanced rest with your babe.
- Lowers risk of breast and ovarian cancer!
- Serves as partial birth control. The hormones used to create breast milk can also prevent ovulation. But this is not a foolproof method, so ask your doc about progesterone-only birth control pills, the IUD, or other forms of birth control that do not release estrogen into your system. Or you could go the old school route and buy some condoms.
- Sucks away the excess weight! Producing breast milk requires boo-coo calories, causing your appetite to reach football-player zone while you lose weight. It's amazing. Eat when you're hungry (no dieting! — you don't need it), and nosh on a variety of flavors, helping to ensure that your baby will have a more versatile palate. Make sure you combine all that food with ample water so the good times keep flowing.
- Makes life easier and more affordable. Your breasts are nourishment on the go; no need to sanitize or heat them up. This ready-made perk is especially beneficial in areas without reliable water sources; the mother's body filters the water used for breast milk, ensuring women can feed their babies without fear of contamination.
- Encourages bonding! There are few emotional tastes sweeter than cradling your baby against your chest and gazing into his eyes while he receives ideal nutrition from you. Baby will likely be staring right back at you during this time. This eye contact and touch releases the aforementioned love hormone, oxytocin, in both of you, and

it fires synapses in Baby's brain, setting him up for a lifetime of awesomeness.

Early Challenges (Or…Opportunities!)

Breastfeeding can suck. But there are ways to make the sucking suck a little less. Having a general idea of how the heck to do it, what to expect, and tricks to try (like squirting your milk on your own nipples and letting it dry) will make your transition into the whole feeding-a-human-from-your-body thing a lot easier.

- **How to do it?** Wash your hands, sit in a comfortable position with your back supported, release the nipple, and pull Baby close to your body (see specific positions described below). Now, touch your nipple to Baby's lips to encourage her to open her mouth, then put your nipple all the way in her mouth until she's latched. You'll know she's latched and receiving milk when her lips are pouted out and almost entirely covering your areola. You should be hearing her swallowing, not smacking.

- **Soreness:** Breastfeeding shouldn't be painful, but it may be a bit uncomfortable in the beginning. If you don't feel that your baby is properly latched on and you're experiencing pain, take him off the breast and try to latch him on again, preferably in a different position. Don't limit breastfeeding if you're feeling discomfort; this could cause a clogged milk duct, which is a whole other breed of discomfort. But do call a lactation consultant and ask for a consultation ASAP. And go topless! Allowing breast milk to dry on the nipple is very soothing and can prevent or heal cracked nipples.

  If one or both of your breasts are red and hot to the touch, you could have a bacterial infection called *mastitis*. You can and should continue to breastfeed, but you should immediately alert your care provider to receive the proper medication.

- **Engorgement:** A few days after birth, you may feel like you've got rock-hard breast implants. Good news: your mature milk is in! Your mature milk will be greater in volume than colostrum, but it will have fewer antibodies. Mature breast milk (now more "milky" in color) also has a higher fat content, helping Baby to develop those cushy rolls. To soften the stony boobs initially created by this milk, apply a warm washcloth to each breast. This too will pass (after a day or two). If your baby has trouble latching on to the engorged breast, self-express (squeeze out some milk with your hand) and try again. If you're worried or are having trouble breastfeeding, call a lactation consultant.

- **Letdowns and leaking:** When you feel a tingling sensation ripple through your breasts (occasionally laced with a slight burning), your milk ducts are filling. When this letdown occurs, find your baby, or a tissue (or ten). If a mouth isn't there to receive the milk, it will eventually push its way out, causing a blob of wetness to bloom from your nipple and soaking your shirt or mattress. (And if it's really pumping it may leak down to your underwear — true story.) When your body eventually syncs up and settles into a rhythm with Baby, you'll notice less leaking, and letdowns will happen only when your baby calls out for a boob.

- **Frequency of feedings:** The feeding needs of a newborn can fluctuate as much as the timing on their diaper blowouts; you never know when it's going to happen, but you better honor it with action when it does. Newborns need a fat helping of on-demand feeding in the first few months of life; they're figuring out the whole "how to be alive" thing and require the nourishment and comfort of breast-feeding to help them assimilate. They'll likely settle into a feeding pattern after a while, but for now, let them eat whenever they seem hungry. Trying to force a feeding schedule too early can slam an unnecessary hammer of frustration down on you and Baby both. And how do you know when to stop a feeding sesh? When Baby seems satisfied and stops on his own, *or* you have to pee really badly. If you need to unlatch baby for whatever reason, insert your finger into the corner of his mouth until you feel him release; this can be especially helpful if Baby ever bites you. Yay!

- **How to know if Baby is getting enough milk:** You'll know your baby received enough milk if she acts satiated after feedings (that is, she's asleep, or not yelling at you) and has six to eight wet diapers, and two to five bowel movements, each day. This number may drop within a few weeks after birth. Trust that your body will produce the exact amount of milk your baby needs.

- **How will you feel?** Breastfeeding will make you hungry, thirsty, and tired *if* you don't nourish yourself with consistent healthy food and a constantly available supply of water and don't allow yourself to rest when your body asks you to. For many women, breastfeeding causes them to require even deeper self-nurturing than pregnancy did; you'll be eating the same diet, but likely more of everything. You may notice an instantaneous thirst the moment you begin a feeding, and the oxytocin that flows as you begin each nursing session will urge your body to sink into the surface below. Don't fight your body's prompts during this time — flow with them, knowing that the best thing you can do for your baby is to care for the body that nourishes them.

- **It's weird!** Yes, it's initially strange to have a little human suck on your nipples to get food. But it will eventually become less strange, so much so that you'll eventually forget what it was like to *not* have your boobs serve as a pantry and fridge. Just think of breastfeeding as a weird miracle of the natural world that you're lucky enough to be a part of.

Positions

In this section you'll find descriptions of the most common breastfeeding positions. Try them all out, being gentle with yourself in the process. They may feel unnatural on the first few tries but will get easier with practice.

- **Cradle hold:** This is the most common and easiest for most women. Place your baby horizontally along your body, right under your breasts, with his face, stomach, and knees facing you. Toy around with where his lower arm seems most comfortable. Cradle his head in the crook of your arm, and support his body with one or both of your forearms (prop up your arms with pillows or the armrests of a chair). Position his head so his mouth is aligned with your nipple. Ensure that your back is supported and you're not hunching over.

- **Side by side:** This position is a primary reason I wasn't a raging mombie (mommy zombie) the first few months of Hudson's life; it allowed me to get some sleep. Lie on your side with pillows supporting your back, head, and neck and one or two pillows between your knees. The idea is to keep your back and hips in a straight line. I recommend purchasing a contoured foam pillow that fully supports the groove of your neck. Now get Baby in there. While lying on your side, position Baby so she's also lying on her side and facing you, with her mouth parallel to your bottom nipple. With the hand of your bottom arm, pull in her body so it's touching yours and guide her mouth to your nipple. If Baby needs to be slightly elevated to comfortably reach your nipple, place a thin (nothing too cushy), folded blanket under her head.
- **Handbag hold:** If you have twins and plan on feeding them at the same time, this is the position for you. If you've had a cesarean birth and don't want little feet kicking the site of your incision, this is the position for you. Tuck Baby under your arm, like an adorable handbag, on the side you'll be nursing him on. Position his body so it's facing you, align his nose with your nipple, and ensure his feet are pointing toward your back. If he's nursing on your right side, slide your right arm under his left arm and hold his head, guiding it toward the nipple. Support his body with a pillow.
- **Whatever works for you:** As long as you and your baby are comfortable, she's able to easily breathe, and she's procuring milk, you're doing great. There is no *wrong* nursing position. Tinker around until you find your sweet (milky) spots. With all positions, ensure your body is fully supported by sitting in a comfortable chair (with stool) or propping yourself up with pillows.

Lactation Consultants

If in doubt, call a lactation consultant. These boob gurus exist for a reason: breastfeeding can be hard, and expert support can significantly help. If you're giving birth in a hospital, a lactation consultant will likely visit you there. If you're having a birth center or home birth, your midwife will set up a home visit with a lactation consultant; confirm this with your care provider.

During the visit the lactation consultant will observe you and Baby breast-feeding and will make suggestions to improve the latch and your comfort. They'll also be available to answer questions, offer moral support, provide breastfeeding nutrition and hydration advice, give you fun facts about breastfeeding, and assist you in the art of pumping.

Your time with a consultant is not the time to be proud; don't pretend you're comfortable and knowledgeable about breastfeeding if you don't actually feel that way. Utilize these services by asking every dang question you can muster, and allow the consultant to get up close and personal with you and Baby while you're breastfeeding. Modesty is the killer of support in this situation. Make sure you pay attention while they're talking, and ask for clarification if there is anything you don't understand.

I met with a lactation consultant before my son was born. She was amazing and gave me so much helpful information — which I didn't retain at the time because I was too busy pretending like I already knew everything she was telling me when I didn't. Allow yourself to be vulnerable and sponge-like during this visit.

You are not limited to one visit with a lactation consultant; call on their services as often as you need until you settle into your new role as Lactator. It's likely your breastfeeding practices and confidence will improve each time you meet with a pro.

Pumping

If you thought breastfeeding was weird, just wait until you strap a sucking machine onto your nips. But the weirdness is worth it — pumping allows you to save and store milk so other people can feed your baby when you need to go back to work, or just want a frigging second to yourself. I've also found pumped milk to be a blessing from the Road Trip Gods when my car-seat-strapped baby was wailing, and unstrapping my own seat belt to lean over him and nurse would be frowned upon by Highway Patrol.

Here are a few considerations to help you navigate the land of noisy boob-suckers:

- **Ask a lactation consultant for pump brand advice:** The Milk Masters know what's up when it comes to artificial milk suckers, so ask them for help. Before making a recommendation they'll ask you what your budget is, how often you plan to pump, how you plan to store the milk, and other questions that will help them help you settle on the ideal pump.

- **Follow the instructions, or ask for help:** When you first use the pump, ask your lactation consultant to come over to assist you in assembly and first use, or meticulously follow the instructions to minimize hassle. Because I skimmed over my instructions, I didn't put in a crucial piece of the pump and spent two pump sessions thinking my pump was a dud (or my boobs were). It is also essential to follow the hygiene and care suggestions that come with your pump to minimize that chance of bacteria ruining the milk.

- **Find the time of day that works best:** There will likely be a time of day that you have a major letdown — mine was around 7:00 AM, when my son was still asleep (and had not drained me) but my milk ducts were ready for him. I would trick them, and hook them up to the pump. If time constraints prevent you from pumping at the time when you have the biggest backlog of milk, you can train your breasts to give it up during the time of day that works best for you. For example, if you have a lunch break at 1:00 PM, find a private space to pump during that time. It may take a few days for your breasts to start flowing at that time, but flow they will; just stick with it.

- **Look at a photo of your baby:** If you're having trouble getting the milk out, look at a photo of your baby to encourage a letdown. Even better, watch a video of your baby fussing or crying. Your body is programmed to let down milk when it senses your baby is in need of comfort; use this programming to your benefit.

- **Let the baby help:** If the pump doesn't offend your baby, you can nurse him on one breast while you pump the other.

- **Distract yourself:** Waiting for your boobs to start cooperating with the pump can be similar to the whole water boiling situation. What's more, if you're feeling antsy waiting for the milk to come, the hormones produced by these nerves could inhibit the flow of milk. Geesh! To bypass this obstacle, distract yourself by watching TV, surfing social media, or napping. (This is possible with practice; I once woke up from a sitting-up nap with twelve ounces of bagged milk strapped to my breasts.)

• **Store milk in small batches, in freezer bags:** You can collect milk in bottles or in freezer bags, specifically made for breast milk, that you can attach to your pump; I recommend the latter. Once milk is pumped it is good for three to four hours in a warm room, four to six hours at room temperature, twenty-four hours in a cooler with freezer packs, three to eight days in the fridge, and six to twelve months in the freezer. Once prepared, bottles of pumped milk are best finished in one sitting. To avoid having to throw out pumped milk (a.k.a. "maternal torture"), use the aforementioned freezer bags to collect milk in small batches, two to five ounces to start. Then, feed your baby from these small servings until you determine how much milk she usually requires in one feeding.

> **EXTRA TIPS:** *Store the bags flat in your freezer so you can stack them and take up less space. Write the date the milk was pumped on the bag and use milk from oldest to newest.*

• **Avoid offering artificial nipples for the first four weeks:** If a newborn tastes the sweet ease of an artificial nipple before they've mastered the trick of getting your real nipples flowing, they could become confused and decide to start flicking your nipples instead of sucking them. Wait at least four weeks after birth, or until breastfeeding is firmly established, before you offer Baby a bottle of pumped milk.

A Few More Things to Know about Pumped Milk

• It's normal for milk to separate into two layers while in the fridge (cream rises to the top). Just swirl the bottle to mix it up.
• The color, consistency, and smell of your milk will vary based on your diet.
• Thawed milk is good in the fridge for twenty-four hours; do not refreeze it.

- To thaw frozen milk, leave it in the fridge overnight or place it in a bowl of warm (not boiling) water for twenty minutes.
- Milk is not spoiled unless it smells very bad or tastes sour.
- Never microwave milk.

From Her Heart to Yours

I wasn't afraid of contractions, or pushing, or the "ring of fire" — I was afraid of breastfeeding. I was afraid my body would fail me and not produce milk. I was afraid my baby wouldn't be able to figure it out. I was afraid my boobs would turn off my husband if milk was leaking out of them. I hired a lactation consultant and doula/hypnotherapist before my son was born to relieve my dread of the whole lactating bosom thing. I practiced different holds on dolls with the support of my lactation consultant, then did three breastfeeding-specific fear-release sessions with my doula and went to a breastfeeding support class where I saw other nervous moms successfully breastfeeding. I even strapped on the pump I purchased. (It tickled! And terrified my husband.)

I moved into childbirth more excited than fearful about the prospect of breastfeeding and ended up having one of those insanely beautiful moments where my newborn wiggled up my chest and found my nipple on his own. A week later, my boobs were cracked and bleeding, and I was crying, but I knew to call my lactation consultant, who came over and assisted me in assisting myself to heal. Ask for help!

— *J. K., Austin, Texas*

RIDDLE: I'm the most common breastfeeding position. What's my first name?

Go to **YourSereneLife.wordpress.com/chapter-twenty** and use the one-word riddle answer as your offer code to download the relaxation recording for this chapter!

CALL TO PLEASURE

- Meditate on all the health benefits breastfeeding holds for you and your baby, allowing yourself to feel proud for committing to something that will so wholly support both your health and your baby's.
- Call a lactation consultant! (Ideally, before you have the baby). Ask them all your questions and don't leave their side until you feel more confident about the act of breastfeeding. Call them back as often as you need, especially when you start breastfeeding a real baby.
- If you plan to pump, buy a pump and supplies with the support of a lactation consultant.
- Create a pumping schedule that suits your body's rhythm.
- Be really nice to yourself through the journey of getting comfortable with breastfeeding. It can be hard, and you don't have to navigate it by yourself. And holy moly, your body is making milk!

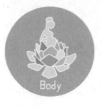

CHAPTER TWENTY-ONE

POSTPARTUM:
My Body Does *What* after Birth?!

JUST BREATHE: *Inhale a hearty dose of healing light to a slow count of eight, then hold for three, envisioning your cells sucking up all this healing. Then slowly exhale to a count of eight, envisioning all pain and tension flowing out of you. Repeat often.*

Movies lie. They mean well, but they lie. Giving birth does not tap you with a wand that transforms you back to pre-pregnancy form. The process your body moves through is more like a slope: you start at zero, the state of your pre-pregnancy body, and slowly climb up the slope, growing to accommodate the human expanding in your womb. You then reach one hundred, childbirth, and then gradually slide back down the slope, possibly returning to zero, or maybe just settling into a gorgeous ten.

Even if you return back to your pre-pregnancy weight, know that your body will never be exactly the same, and that's awesome. The reshaping that your body goes through during pregnancy, birth, and beyond also re-shapes your mind and spirit, molding you into a new whole-being who re-sembles your old Self, but is now layered in greater self-love, a knowingness of your unbreakable strength, and bigger boobs.

What to Expect When Your Womb Becomes Vacant

Few women are prepared for the belly bulge, unpredictable hormonal surges, and soreness that are knit into the postpartum experience. No longer having a baby in your womb yet having a body that is vastly different than your prebaby body is difficult for many new moms. We all experience a postpartum shift in our sense of body identity that is, frankly, jarring. This chapter guides you through the physical changes that anchor you in your new postpartum world, and it encourages you to look at these physical changes with appreciation, instead of judgment. Learning to love your changing maternal body is grounding and empowering in ways that will transform you.

We'll focus on what you can expect with your postbirth body: lochia, swelling, hemorrhoids, hair loss, soreness, belly pooch, and a feeling of instability in your bladder and uterus. Symptoms will vary depending on the type of labor you had, and any preexisting medical conditions you may have.

Lochia

Lochia, a.k.a. "postpartum discharge," usually comes in the form of blood and tissue shed from the uterus and bacteria. This bleeding and discharge will be similar to a *very* heavy period the first few days postpartum, and then thin out to (mostly) bloodless discharge about ten days postpartum, with possible spotting for a few weeks thereafter. This normal loss of blood isn't dangerous, as the amount of blood in your body increases by 50 percent during pregnancy. Note that if you've been lying down for a while, allowing the blood to collect, you may see blood clots in your pad after you stand up and go to the bathroom. Normal.

If you notice an increase in lochia after physically exerting yourself, or just walking to the mailbox, take this as a sign to rest. Let your flow of lochia be your reminder to take it easy. "I'm sorry I can't put in that load of laundry — because...lochia."

Where Does the Blood Come From?

When the placenta breaks away from the uterus, it leaves behind open blood vessels that bleed into the uterus. As the uterus contracts, the blood vessels will begin to close and the bleeding will subside. If you had a vaginal tear during delivery, it's normal for that site to bleed as well.

Because I didn't know any of this, I thought my vagina was the star of a horror movie when I just kept bleeding (and bleeding and bleeding) the first few days postpartum. Come to find out it was just the star of a basic documentary about the normal behavior of a postpartum vagina.

How Much Is Too Much?

Your care provider will give you guidelines about how much blood is normal. Alert your care provider if the blood is still bright red four days postpartum and is not getting any lighter. You should also call for support if your lochia has a putrid odor or you're experiencing fever or chills. If you completely saturate a pad in one hour, or have a blood clot bigger than a golf ball, call for care immediately.

What You'll Need

The *biggest* pads you can find, and even bigger underwear to strap them on. (I recommend buying a big pack of comfortable sexy-less panties.) For the love of your vagina, *no* tampons. As the blood tapers off, you can downgrade to smaller pads. You'll also need to set reminders to empty your bladder as it may be less sensitive after the insane ride it was just on — it may not be as proficient to alerting you that it's at full capacity. A full bladder can cause urinary problems and prevent your uterus from properly contracting.

Swelling (a.k.a. "Postpartum Edema")

Please let the fact that you'll be fairly swollen following birth bring you comfort. I thought my swelling was made of fat, and it made me sad. This swelling is not fat. It is a combo of excess blood, hormonal changes, and retained fluid, and it should be gone in about a week after birth.

How Much Is Too Much?

If the swelling does not subside after one week, grows in intensity, or is accompanied by symptoms such as breathing problems, extreme discomfort, or low urine output, call the doc.

How to Soothe It

Eat meals rich in protein and potassium (lots of fresh fruits and veggies), avoid processed foods full of sodium, drink dandelion tea, get the blood flowing by walking around, sit back and elevate your feet above the level of your heart, have your partner give you a leg and foot massage, soak your feet, sit in a cool room (heat intensifies swelling), maintain good posture, avoid clothing or accessories that prevent blood flow, and drink water, and then more water, to flush out the fluid your body is holding on to.

Hemorrhoids

These little bastards are made of hemorrhoidal blood vessels pushing out the anus. Yay! If you didn't develop hemorrhoids before birth from the pressure of your growing uterus and possible constipation, pushing your baby out will usually do the trick. Hemorrhoids often range in sensation from itchy to painful, and range in size from raisin to grape — Yum.

How to Make Them Suck Less

Because hemorrhoids are as much fun as they sound, utilize the following "butt pain alleviators": medicated wipes after bowel movements, cold compresses on the scene of the crime (up the comfort level by saturating the compress in witch hazel), soaking your butt in a warm sitz bath, sitting on a donut, medicated hemorrhoid cream (ask your care provider for a recommendation), and a knowingness that they will likely go away on their own after they've had their fun.

How to Avoid Inviting More Hemorrhoids to the Party

You can prevent more hemorrhoids from poking out by eating a fiber-rich diet (or ask your care provider to recommend a stool softener) so your bowel movements are easy breezy. Use the bathroom as soon as you feel the urge, and avoid pushing too hard. In addition, continue your Kegels to ensure the muscles around your rectum are strong and less likely to let any unruly blood vessels escape.

When to Call for Help

Although rectal bleeding during a bowel movement can be normal when hemorrhoids are at your potty party, you should still alert your care provider if you notice any blood in your stools.

Hair Loss

You can't have your baby and keep your extra hair too. During pregnancy, estrogen causes more hair to grow and less to fall out. When estrogen levels drop after birth, the excess hair will begin falling out. The good news is you won't go bald; the hair loss will eventually stop six to twelve months after birth, and you'll likely be left with your pre-pregnancy hair — and a clogged shower drain.

What to Do

While you can't prevent your hormones from having their way with your hair follicles, you can work with them. Donning a classic "mom cut" will help to hide the appearance of your thinning hair and be easier to maintain. Or do as I did and wear your long hair in a wet (sometimes greasy) bun for the first year of Baby's life.

Marathon Soreness

Twenty-four to forty-eight hours after giving birth vaginally, your muscles and joints will likely feel like you ran a marathon. Even if you didn't move around much during labor, every fiber of your body was put through intense exertion during labor, and that equals mega-soreness. It is normal. It will go away after a few days. It can be alleviated.

What to Do

First, have your partner book you a postpartum massage — you have never deserved a professional massage more. You can also take warm baths, filling each tub with the following ingredients: 1½ cup Epsom salt, 6 tablespoons baking soda, 6 tablespoons witch hazel, 3 tablespoons olive oil, 16–24 drops of lavender essential oil, and 16–24 drops of chamomile essential oil. Utilize hugs *and* drugs. No need to be a martyr — ask your care provider about any over-the-counter medication you can take (usually acetaminophen) to calm down your discomfort. And stay hydrated; a lack of water can exaggerate the soreness in your muscles.

When to Call for Help

If the soreness does not subside after a few days, grows in intensity, or is more painful than uncomfortable, tell your care provider. If you experience none of this but just want a professional to tell you that everything you're feeling is normal, call your care provider.

Belly Pooch

For a few weeks after birth, you may experience a saggy bloat that makes you look like you're about five or six months pregnant. This will last until your uterus shrinks back down to pre-pregnancy size and hormonal shifts cause the swelling to drain away through sweat, urine, and vaginal secretions. Because the pooch is made up of an additional goody, fat, you'll probably still be left with a little two-to-three-months-pregnant pooch after the swelling drains and the uterus deflates. The excess fat doesn't have to be a permanent resident, but don't be too hasty in throwing it out; it is a building block of the milk your body is producing.

Your belly's embellishments — the dark vertical line called the *linea nigra* and possibly stretch marks — will also fade after about twelve months (maybe longer).

What to Do

Be gentle with yourself, putting more focus on what your body can do (e.g., growing, birthing, and feeding a baby) than on what it looks like. In addition, breastfeed as often as your baby wants. Breastfeeding can burn up to five hundred calories a day, helping to suck that cute pooch right out of you. To support your belly-trimming efforts, eat a healthy diet, rich with whole foods grown from the earth; drink more water than you think you need;

and slowly ease back into light exercise (under the supervision of your care provider). Avoid a strict diet, as it could inhibit your milk production and cause fatigue and negative shifts in your mood.

When to Call for Support

The transformed postpartum body instills pride in some, and shame in others. If you feel frustrated with your body, you can call in the support of a nutritionist or trainer. But the most powerful support may be in the form of a therapist who can help you learn to love your new body. When we feel unconditional love for our bodies, they oftentimes organically find their way back to their ideal size and shape. If your pooch is hard, swollen, and painful, call your care provider.

You Feel Like Your Uterus and Bladder Are Falling Out

Yes, you may feel like your lower-hanging organs are sagging down and attempting to plop out of you, especially when you're having a poop. But they won't, I promise. Your expanding uterus pushed around your organs, and they're now trying to find their way home. While this feels weird, it's normal. In addition, your pelvic floor muscles may have weakened from the strain of childbirth and the flood of relaxin (the relaxing hormone), causing your uterus and bladder to droop down.

What to Do

Pelvic floor exercises! Lots of them. Maintaining strong pelvic floor muscles before, during, and after pregnancy will help to ensure your organs have a nice foundation to sit on and do not start sagging. For a pelvic floor exercise recap, see page 56.

When to Call for Support

If you feel excessive pressure and discomfort on and in your pelvic floor, have lower abdominal pain or strong aching in your back, or see or feel a bulge in your vaginal area, call your care provider. You could possibly be experiencing uterine prolapse. Showing up to all your postpartum checkups will also help to ensure everything is properly moving back into place.

Getting to Know Your Postpartum Body

While you're technically in the same body you were in pre-pregnancy, the inner and outer landscape of that body has shifted. How your body now responds to food, sex, exercise, clothes, and more is likely different. While these changes are initially jarring, they can be reframed in a way that allows you to celebrate them, instead of mourning their presence.

To do this, look at yourself in the mirror (clothing optional!) and, out loud, tell your body how grateful you are to it for growing, birthing, and now nursing your child. Continue to offer your reflection messages of love until you perceive the body you're viewing as strong and beautiful. To get a deeper understanding of what's happening beneath your skin, get chummy with your medical care provider, asking them all The Questions about all The Things. Getting to know the new inner and outer workings of your transformed body will help you feel more at home in it.

Ask All Your Questions at Your Six-Week Checkup

Who cares about judge-y labels like "hypochondriac" or "paranoid" — if you're concerned (or just curious) about something you're experiencing, call your care provider for answers and support. Every time a question pops up between birth and your postpartum checkup, write it down, then ask your care provider. Yes, the internet knows a lot, but it doesn't know your exact medical history. Your care provider does; ask them, not Google.

Here are a few questions to jump-start you: "When can I start having sex?" (Yes, you are allowed to lie to your partner and give them a number larger than the one your care provider gives you.) "What are my birth control options?" "Where is my mind?" Please don't be modest with your questions; I promise your care provider has heard far stranger.

From Her Heart to Yours

I felt like a thin piece of broken glass that had been pieced back together with drugs and sutures after my daughter's forty-two-hour birth. Going to the bathroom was totally disgusting, what with the blood and what felt like giant pimples poking out of my bum. Yuck. I didn't know all of this was normal. My horror came from a place of "not knowing." I felt fragile and, frankly, appalled with my body because I was unaware it was doing exactly what it was supposed to be doing. A panicked call to my care provider's cell at 6 AM on a Sunday is what finally assuaged my crazy. In gory detail I described everything coming out of my body. She asked a few questions (about smells and such) and calmly told me that my body was "a champ" at navigating postpartum symptoms, acting exactly as it was supposed to. My body was a champ! Hearing this shifted my perception of my body's postbirth display, and I began to feel a sense of awe for my body, not repulsion.

— *P. G., San Antonio, Texas (a total champ)*

RIDDLE: I'm the vaginal discharge you can expect a visit from after birth. Who am I?

Go to **YourSereneLife.wordpress.com/chapter-twenty-one** and use the one-word riddle answer as your offer code to download the relaxation recording for this chapter!

CALL TO PLEASURE

- Talk to your care provider about what to expect from your body after birth, and what "red flags" to look out for. If a red flag does pop up, don't hesitate to call your care provider.
- Avoid using the internet as your source of information. You'll likely find more "worst-case scenario" advice than support that pertains to your specific situation.
- Allow complete nurturing of your body for the first forty days after birth. Accept all forms of help, sleep as often as you can, eat what you feel like, sit in a dark room with your baby and watch your favorite movie — do what feels good to *you*.

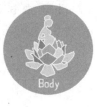

CHAPTER TWENTY-TWO

ODD YET COMMON BABY CARE QUESTIONS:
Poop Color, Spit-Up, and Beyond!

JUST BREATHE: *Inhale a stream of all-encompassing love to a slow count of ten. As you exhale to the same count, imagine Baby being filled and surrounded by this potent love.*

The bodily fluids, abstract facial expressions, and indecipherable sounds that an infant produces can be alarming. You may be secretly terrified that you'll miss an important cue from your baby, or make a misstep that will have dire consequences.

As you move through this chapter, your fears will be soothed as you gain answers to the common questions new moms have, yet seldom ask. Your trust in your maternal intuition will grow as you realize how resilient and strong babies are, and how motivated they are to communicate their needs. In this chapter, I will discuss how to stay relaxed and present so you can best receive messages and information from your baby and tune in to the powerful mother-baby connection that will become the lifelong foundation of this beautiful relationship.

My hope is that you'll be less grossed out by all the stuff that comes out of your baby's mouth and booty (and the stuff that grows in her crevices) because you'll know her little body is just doing as nature instructed.

What's the Lowdown on Poop?

Babies are first-class poopers — moving that matter through their bowels quicker than it takes them to empty your boob, and sometimes pooping so hard and fast it blasts up their back. Diaper blowouts = mega-fun. Because baby poop comes in many colors, consistencies, and amounts, it's important to know the difference between poop that seems alarming but is normal, and poop that seems alarming because it's a sign of something that requires medical attention. Here's your guide to what comes out your baby's booty:

- **Frequency:** Babies vary in how often they poo, with some moving it through after every meal, and some only eliminating a few times a week. Newborns often have a bowel movement after every feeding (ten-ish times a day), and after three to six weeks settle into a routine that consists of fewer, but more predictable, movements.

- **Consistency:** Because Baby will be consuming only liquids the first six months of life, his poop should be relatively soft, even liquid, in consistency. If the poop is coming out hard, it could be a sign of constipation, which warrants a call to the pediatrician.

- **Meconium:** Motor oil poo! This is the sticky, dark-green or black, tar-like poop your baby will eliminate the first few days after birth. This concoction is made up of skin cells, goodies ingested in utero, mucus, and amniotic fluid. Shockingly, it doesn't have an odor, so do a visual check of Babe's diaper on a regular basis to ensure she's not sitting in her own goo (some babies don't mind the feeling and will not alert you when their diaper is soiled).

- **Breastfed poop:** If it looks like your baby's bowels deposited a helping of split pea soup after your milk comes in, they are doing great. Exclusively breastfed poop is often yellow or green in color, the consistency of mushy soup (sometimes nearing a broth consistency), could have cottage cheese–looking chunks in it, and is possibly sprinkled with what looks like mustard seeds. All normal. And as an extra kiss from the Breastfeeding Gods, it doesn't smell like much more than mild curry. There is no set criteria for "healthy breastfed baby poop" — its color and consistency will likely vary, depending on what you're eating.

- **Not-getting-enough-fatty-milk poop:** If baby delivers bright-green, foamy poop into her diaper she may not be breastfeeding long enough, causing her to consume more of the watery foremilk, and less of the fatty hindmilk. Encourage her to drain each breast during feedings, and rouse her awake by rubbing her cheek if she conks out after forty-five seconds on the teat.
- **Formula-fed poop:** Formula-fed poop is often similar to peanut butter in color and consistency and is a bit more odorous than breast milk poo.
- **Solid-food poop:** When you decide to introduce solid foods (sometime after Baby's six-month birthday), his poop will likely become darker and thicker — and smellier! If you occasionally see what looks like undigested food in the poop, that's normal. If you see undigested food in every diaper, tell your doc as this could be a sign that Baby's intestines are having trouble absorbing nutrients.
- **Constipation:** If it looks like little pebbles have been dropped in your baby's diaper, she's probably constipated. This can happen when you make the switch to solid food, or when Baby has sensitivity to the milk or formula she's being given. Let a professional know if the pebble-poop lasts for more than a few diapers, or is accompanied by blood.
- **Diarrhea:** Baby diarrhea is almost entirely liquid and often comes in the hue of yellow, brown, or green. This is often the stuff "diaper blowouts" are made of. While some diarrhea can be normal, it can lead to dehydration, and if it is consistent it may be a possible sign of infection. If your baby has diarrhea over a period of a few days or fills more than two or three diapers with diarrhea in one day, call the doctor.
- **Warning signs:** If your baby is acting unusually fussy and you can't soothe him with your normal methods (e.g., breastfeeding, burping, rocking, shushing, diaper changing, yodeling, etc.), it could be a sign of gastrointestinal issues. There is no need for serious alarm, but because tummy issues are zero fun for all involved, call the pediatrician. If you notice a change in your baby's bowel movements,

P.S. *Finding your baby's poop (or toots) cute is not weird. I was stoked each time my baby had a BM because it meant his body was working.*

accompanied by other symptoms (e.g., fever, rash, loss of appetite, abnormal fussiness, etc.), alert the baby doc. If you see bright-red blood in the diaper, this could be a sign of infection, hemorrhoids, allergy, or other potential issues that need to be treated under the care of a medical professional. (If the poop is so dark it's almost black, it's digested blood that was likely picked up from a cracked and bleeding nipple and is nothing to worry about). As a general rule, call your baby's doctor if the poop ever seems alarming to you.

Is Projectile Spit-Up Normal?

Yes, usually. And yes, it's okay if you're completely horrified by it.

Because Baby's digestive system is still figuring things out, it's common for a bit of milk to come back up after feedings, and sometimes a whole lotta milk comes back out, à la The Exorcist. If Baby is gaining weight, doesn't seem bothered by the spit-up, and isn't fussier than usual, you probably don't have anything to be concerned with. But follow your intuition. If your baby's spit-up worries you, or she projectile vomits more than once each day, let your baby's care provider know.

Skin Care

How Do I Know if My Baby Has a Diaper Rash? And How Do I Handle It?

A diaper rash is made of red, inflamed skin on your baby's bottom, and it's considered a diaper rash caused by yeast if the rash is accompanied by little red dots. If your baby has consistent diaper rashes, consider changing his diaper more often, switching the type of diapers or wipes you use, or experimenting with eliminating certain foods from your diet that may irritate Baby's skin when it is introduced via fecal matter. If you try all these methods and the rashes keep on coming, ask for your doctor's help.

Diaper Rash Care

Squirt some breast milk on it! Breast milk is a miracle cure for many nasty ailments, like pinkeye, cracked nipples, and booty rashes. Dry off your baby's bum, squirt and gently spread breast milk onto it (you can self-express some from your breast), and allow your babe to go diaper-less for a while. The idea is to let the area breathe, while being nourished by a healing natural ointment. If you're not breastfeeding, coconut oil is a great alternative treatment.

When Do I Bathe Baby?

A newborn shouldn't be submerged in water until their umbilical cord stump has fallen off. Before the stump has dislodged from the belly button, you can wipe out your baby's crevices (which may grow yummy cheese from a buildup of milk) with a wet washcloth. After the stump falls off, you can bathe Baby a few times a week (or just stick with the washcloth crevice baths), making sure not to dry out her skin by bathing her too much or using a harsh soap (warm water will do just fine). When you decide to "full-on" bathe, remember that Baby will be slippery, so use a baby bath that will support her full body and submerge her in only a few inches of water, being sure to have a hand and both eyes on her at all times. *Never leave Baby unattended in a bath, even for a second!* Before your baby is born it's good policy to set your water heater below 120 degrees Fahrenheit, and always check the water temp with your hand before placing your baby into it.

Cord Stump Care

Keep that sucker dry. To properly fall off (which usually happens between two and three weeks after birth), the stump of Baby's umbilical cord needs to have a dry and clean environment. Keep the area around the stump clean with a wipe or damp washcloth, taking care not to wipe the actual stump, and always fold the front of the diaper in toward your baby's belly to prevent urine from getting on the cord stump; the top of the diaper should be under the cord stump, not covering it. The stump will turn black-ish when it's about to fall off.

Sleep

Where Should Baby Sleep?

Aw, heck, you'll have to decide this one on your own. As long as Baby is on his back and away from items that could suffocate him (e.g., fluffy blankets, pillows, crib bumper, or stuffed animals), the best place for him to sleep is where you both feel most comfortable. If neither of you can sleep when you're apart, consider safe cosleeping options. If you wake each other up with every flick of a finger, consider different beds in the same room. You'll likely need to use some trial and error (or "sleep" and "no-sleep" nights) to find your sleepy sweet spot. Cosleeping always worked best for my family, but I know other mamas whose babies couldn't settle when sharing a bed with the parents. Do what works best for *you and Baby*, not the nosy people who ask you about your sleeping arrangement then tell you what you "should" be doing.

Should Baby Sleep on Her Back?

Yes! Always! This significantly reduces the chance of sudden infant death syndrome (SIDS). The only exception is if she's sleeping on your body, or lying sideways to sleepy nurse (in which case you should lie her on her back when she breaks the latch).

Why Do Newborns Make Weird Sleep Sounds?

Newborns don't "sleep like babies" — they sleep like newborns who want to eat every two to four hours, and maybe more. On average, newborns sleep 16.5 hours per day (with huge variations!) and spend half of that time in rapid eye movement (REM) mode. During REM, Baby is in a light and active sleep, commonly making whimpers and moans or falling into strange breathing patterns. This irregular breathing is actually pretty regular. Babies have an average rate of forty breaths per minute while awake and may slow to half that during sleep. But that's an average; Baby might take many rapid and shallow breaths over a period of twenty seconds, then take a long pause without any breaths — babies be trippin'. Their breathing eventually becomes less trippy, when the breathing-control center in their brains figures out what's what. Nasal breathing, whistling, and gurgling are also par for the course when it comes to baby sleep. A potential sign of distress that warrants a call to a professional is rapid breathing that stays rapid, consistent flaring of nostrils at the end of breaths, grunting after every breath, or muscles under his ribs or in his neck retracting deeper than usual.

Between REM cycles, your baby will be semi-awake for a moment — usually making a sound that tricks you into thinking he's full-on awake — before falling into the next sleep cycle. Give yourself a few beats before you rush over when hearing what you think is Baby rousing from sleep; he may slip back into his dream.

General Comfort

Is Baby Too Hot? Too Cold?

Imagine not being able to take off your sweater when you're hot, or to put on the fuzzy socks when you're cold. Welcome to the temperature dependence Baby has on you. It's crucial to ensure that your baby isn't getting too hot or too cold. You don't need to be paranoid, but you should keep tabs on her temperature comfort and make adjustments as necessary.

Signs your baby is too hot include feeling hot to the touch (hotter than her norm), sweating, heat rash, restlessness, damp hair, or continued rapid breathing. If the temperature in a space is a nice temperature for you, it's likely fine for Baby. If your baby is dressed in clothing layers and material similar to your own, and you're comfortable, she likely is as well. (The exception is when you're outside in cold temperatures, when you should put a hat on Baby as she loses a significant amount of heat from her head.) If she has a temperature (100.4 degrees Fahrenheit or higher, rectally), let your pediatrician know, especially if your babe has other symptoms. During the winter months keep your baby warm at night, using a wearable blanket rather than a blanket that may collect around her face.

The primary sign that Baby is too cold is if her tummy or chest is cold to the touch. If these areas are chilly and she seems agitated, add a layer of clothing.

In regards to SIDS, it's more dangerous for Baby to sleep in a room that is too hot than too cool; it's more difficult for babies to wake and alert us to something going wrong in their body if they're sedated by heat. The ideal room temp for sleepy time is sixty-nine to seventy-five degrees Fahrenheit.

Should I Massage My Baby?

Yes. Your touch will be one of your newborn's favorite sensations. Take an infant massage course to learn the proper methods for giving your newborn a gentle massage; it will support him in so many ways: relaxing, forging a deeper bond with you, sleeping better, tuning in to his body awareness, feeling loved, boosting his immune system, improving the condition of his skin, enhancing his digestive system, relieving teething discomfort, and more! Infant massages rock — they're affordable and effective and they'll make you feel like you're really doing something to enhance your early experience with Baby. And then, schedule a massage for yourself.

Final Points to Increase Your Peace

Make a List of Questions for Your Pediatrician

There are no stupid questions, Mama! Write down *every* question that comes up and ask them all at your child's next checkup, or call up the doc if your questions can't wait. I don't care if you take two hours of your child's pediatrician's time asking your tome of queries — you deserve to be soothed by accurate information, and they can provide that information.

If in Doubt, Keep Baby Close

If your baby seems "off" in any way, keep her close to you until you can get her in front of a medical professional. Remember that skin-to-skin contact will help her regulate her temperature, breathing, blood pressure and rate, and sense of calm.

Listen to Your Mamawareness

You will be the best barometer for predicting whether your baby is okay or not. Sure, you'll have moments of paranoia, but when you settle into the moment through deep breathing and a still body, you'll likely tap into that wise-mama voice living in your core that will tell you whether all is well or you need to act. Practice moving into this space many times a day (when poop isn't flying); while here, you'll be a Master Radar at picking up on messages from your baby, and tuning in to the powerful mother-baby connection that will become the lifelong foundation of this beautiful relationship.

Remember, Babies Are Tougher Than They Look

Babies are masters of disguise, masking their tough interiors with soft, adorable exteriors. Although Baby needs your almost constant care and attention the first few months following birth, he'll be able to withstand so much more than you ever thought possible. Don't let knowledge of this toughness silence your mamawareness if it's telling you to seek medical attention for your baby, but do let it comfort you when you gaze at his seemingly fragile little body, thinking, "How the heck am I going to get this tiny thing to adulthood?" (or when you accidentally bonk his head when trying to get him into the freaking stroller).

From Her Heart to Yours

Getting the heads-up about "newborn stuff" from books and opinionated acquaintances bolstered my confidence when moving from pregnancy to mothering, but it was nothing compared to the crazy-loud intuition that turned on when my uterus kicked my baby out. Holding her, listening to her, watching her, talking to her, sitting in silence with her, thinking about her, wiping poop off her…every moment of connection we had served to deepen my knowledge of her, and my trust that I knew how to care for her and when to call in support. I had a few moments of "freak out" — calling the on-call doctor at weird hours or sobbing in the shower with a candy bar — but for the most part I was really surprised by my innate ability to mother my unique child.

— *C. R., Lake Tahoe, California (mamawareness master)*

RIDDLE: I'm the black, sticky poop that comes out of your baby the first few days after birth. What's my name?

Go to **YourSereneLife.wordpress.com/chapter-twenty-two** and use the one-word riddle answer as your offer code to download the relaxation recording for this chapter.

CALL TO PLEASURE

- Keep a running list of questions for Baby's pediatrician, and then ask all of them.
- If you're worried, call the medical care provider!
- Nurture yourself — this will result in deeper nurturing of your baby. Take a nap, eat your favorite meal, watch too much Netflix, walk (or just stand) outside, make out with your partner — do what makes you feel like you for a second.
- Breathe through the confusion. It will get easier.

CHAPTER TWENTY-THREE

MOMMY-BABY LOVIN'

Just Breathe: With each deep inhalation feel yourself settling into motherhood, allowing confidence, courage, and strong intuition to flow through you. As you exhale, feel all doubt, regret, and fear pour out of you.

There has never been and never again will be a child just like yours; even though babies are born every day, the birth of your baby is sacred, unique, and extraordinary. Connecting to this unique heart energy of your baby will be a profound experience for you, allowing your internal trapdoor of love to release. Physical nourishment aside, physically and emotionally bonding with your baby is the surest way to build a secure base that will provide your child confidence, support, love, and abundant health for the rest of her life. Developing a harmonic connection with your baby is what it's all about.

In this chapter, I will remind you that your relationship with your rapidly growing and changing baby is fluid and dynamic, and that you have the chance to grow and learn to be a better communicator, better partner, and better parent as you incorporate this new relationship into your family constellation. This chapter will also support you in finding that place that is so deep in yourself there are no words — only love. You have a limited number of vowels and consonants but an unlimited supply of love that will support you in forging an everlasting connection with your child.

The Love Is in the Science

Did you know your baby's scent is custom made to make him irresistible to you? Baby secretes pheromones, the kind of chemicals we secrete to attract a partner, from his nostrils that draw you in for kisses and cuddling. This scent is so appealing to mamas, and so unique to the baby, that many mothers can identify their baby using scent alone. Baby also has a mama-attuned sniffer, able to identify his mother without the need to peek. Your scent (specifically the scent of your breast milk) even has the ability to soothe your baby when you're not physically there to nurture him. So leave behind one of your used shirts and a bottle of your booby nectar when you need to leave Baby in the care of a "not you." Remember, your body is completely on board with helping you fall into the most epic love affair with Baby.

Your brain is in on the action, too. The rewards-processing center of a mother's brain has been proven to light up when she sees a photo of her child, and *really* light up when she sees a photo of Baby smiling. Science tells us how to keep Baby nurtured: Mama does something to make Baby smile, Mama likes Baby's smile and wants more of them, Mama does more stuff to make Baby smile, and around we go. You are prewired to become addicted to your child's happiness, and your child's brain is primed to be positively conditioned by this (mostly) happy environment you will in turn provide for him.

This bonding does more than just shape your baby's early whole-being growth; data are being discovered in the fields of biology, neurology, psychology, and anthropology (to name a few) that back up the belief that a mother's loving care and attention not only support a child's early development but are also drawing the blueprint for how the child will send and receive love well into adulthood.

While some view these strong forces of early bonding as putting a lot of pressure on moms, you can practice viewing it as an opportunity to get a jump on deeply rooting your love into your child so you'll have less work to do when he's older. What do I mean by "less work"? If your child is infused at an early age with the knowing that he is loved and safe, he'll be better able to handle difficult emotions throughout his adolescent years and beyond, be more adventurous (in an "eyes wide open" sort of way) in his life decisions, and feel more comfortable coming to you for guidance. Essentially, the teenage years won't suck as much.

Bonding for Brain Cells

"Make Baby Smart" videos, classical music, baby sign language classes, mini-yoga, and so on — there's a ball pit full of tools available to "turn your offspring into a future Noble Prize–winning astrophysicist." But research is showing that the best way to raise your babe's IQ, and potentially enhance the growth of her hippocampus (the region in the brain that is crucial for memory, reactions to stress, and learning) is tender-loving cuddles, and lots of them. Although bonding is a lifelong opportunity, your baby's brain is busiest in the first two years of life; the processing of information, touch, and development of new skills puts Baby's brain in hyperdrive. Nurturing this process with "in-the-moment" play, interaction, and caressing will strengthen the symphony of synapses taking place in Baby's mind, helping her to reach optimal development.

FUN FACT: *It's believed that all babies are born "prematurely" because their brains need not nine but eighteen months to fully develop. It's only because their heads wouldn't be able to fit through the vag at eighteen months that they're born at nine months. That's why the first nine months after birth are often referred to as exterogestation.*

Bonding for Health

Bonding is just as essential as meeting a baby's physiological needs; it may even affect his physiological needs. Epigenetics — the study of how environmental factors, such as what you consume, how you deal with stress, whether you exercise, and what you breathe in, can physically alter certain genes, turning them "on" or "off" — has shown that how much TLC a baby receives can affect what signals that baby's immature and confused bundle of nerves sends off. The nurturing you provide through activities like skin-to-skin contact, talking, singing, dancing, cooing, and more will help your baby's nerves send off more stable signals, which in turn support him in regulating his sensations of hunger, discomfort, sight, temperature fluctuations, discordant noises, and all the other crazy-new sensations he is being hit with. If your baby has to navigate all this newness without your comfort and guidance, the bombardment of these sensations can cause him immense stress, lowering his immunity. And cells remember — they remember the stress they were exposed to as newbies, which causes them to hold on to the lowered immunity well into adulthood.

Bonding = your enhanced ability to read and respond to Baby's cues = a more stable internal regulation of Baby's needs = less stressor hormones running through Baby's body = a stronger immune system for Baby.

Science backs up the belief that cuddling could minimize the occurrence of physical ailments caused by a weak immune system; premature babies who receive frequent touch gain weight and thrive more than premature babies who are lacking in skin-to-skin contact. These cuddled preemies tend to maintain better temperature control, breathe easier, have more stable heart rates, and have mamas who are able to keep up their milk production.

How to Do It

The best way to achieve these bonding-related health benefits is to "wear" Baby as much as possible, using a comfortable wrap or baby carrier. In addition to a strengthened immune system, Baby's sense of balance and movement will be improved as she feels how you maintain your balance and move throughout the world. (Did you know babies who experience more carry time actually walk sooner than many babies who are left to their own devices?) And most baby carriers allow for hands-free breastfeeding; whipping out your boob and giving Baby a snack while strolling down the produce aisle is a strange kind of wonderful.

Bonding for Adventure

Bonding isn't for sissies — it's for bold individuals willing to (lovingly) kick fear's ass. Receiving potent bonding time with the primary caregiver, even before birth, instills a deep-seated sense of security, confidence, and courageousness in children, who will later grow into secure, confident, and courageous adults. If a human being of any age knows they have a safe haven of love to return to, they will feel more optimistic and sure of their abilities to journey away from this comfort zone, because they know they can always return to replenish.

Babies who are deprived of this critical connection and care from their primary caregiver do not simply "figure it out for themselves" or learn to "deal with it"; instead these children develop a strong yearning for security, care, and comfort and will search for it until it is obtained. It is unlikely that children lacking in loving connection will develop the courage to fully "dive into life" until their primal needs for this connection and love are met. Gift your child with the ability to seek and explore his passions by together building an emotional cocoon of love that will serve as his reservoir of security and "courage recharge station" the rest of his life.

Quality and (Reasonable) Quantity

Babies didn't coin the adage "It's not the quantity but the quality" — they want both when it comes to their bonding time with Mama. When your child is a newborn she can never have too much of you; if she had it her way, she wouldn't just be *with* you, but *on* you (and probably back in you) at all times. You truly are everything to your baby at this time in her life, and she'll let you know that by (vocally) yearning for your almost constant companionship.

Spending an abundant quantity of quality time with your baby is not just a benefit for her, but a life-transforming gift for yourself as well. Learning to slow down and appreciate both the minute and immense beauty in life, and in each other, is pretty special. Don't forget to tell your baby thank you for being the best teacher you'll ever know.

But…it is possible to reach "bonding burnout." So make sure you have occasional breaks from your baby (try using the suggestions listed in chapter 19) so the periods you do spend together are more potent. And find peace in knowing that as your little one grows into a scooter, crawler, and then walker, she will still like her quantity but will start to put more emphasis on the quality, allowing you more freedom to poop by yourself or eat a meal with both hands.

And we don't need to get extreme with the quality, either. If you feel like sitting on the couch and watching television, you can achieve good-enough bonding at the same time by holding your baby on your chest, allowing her to grip and ungrip your fingers as you meditate on how beautiful Thor is.

How to Teach Baby All the Things through Mirroring and Eye Contact

Babies learn through observation and interaction, which is why my toddler smacks my butt every time he walks by me, and calls me a babe before he asks for candy.

No pressure, but your baby will learn almost all his early "ways of being" from you. (Okay, so that's a *little* pressure.) When you exhibit positive actions, emotions, or habits in front of your baby, his brain wakes up and accepts these seeds of information that will later blossom into his ever-evolving character. When you mirror your baby, he learns to trust that his self-expression elicits various responses, and the more your baby learns which expressions garner specific responses, the more he develops the ability to communicate more effectively. When your baby smiles at you, smile back; when your baby giggles, giggle back; when your baby has a fit fest…

Do you feel like a caricature when you're mirroring Baby? I hope so. Your exaggerated enthusiasm is just what he needs. Your mimicking will not offend your sprout, like it probably would your partner or peer. Your animated mirroring will help him become more in tune with his emotional experiences. Take for example, actual mirrors; imagine peering into a tiny hand-held mirror to view how you look, and now imagine peering into a full-length mirror. Which one would provide a more complete image? Your exaggerated mirroring provides your baby with complete feedback on his expressions and corresponding emotions, and enhances his perceptual understanding.

What If You Don't Experience Love at First Sight?

There are many reasons (e.g., postpartum depression, a disappointing birth experience, medications, etc.) why you might not experience the kind of instant love connection with your baby that makes the bonding process easier. But this does not mean your baby can't still benefit from all the goodies mentioned in this chapter. As long as you stay committed to ensuring your baby's needs are met by "faking it till you make it" and supplementing your own love and care with the support of friends and family members, your baby can still be infused with the mental, physical, and spiritual thriving that come with a solid mother-baby bond.

Although there's nothing wrong with you not having an insta-connect with your baby, you probably do want that. Here are a few ways to foster the connection:

- **Are you consuming your daily dose of empathy?** You are not a bad parent if the sight of your baby doesn't immediately melt your heart and transform you into a cooing machine. If you just had a baby come out your vagina, you have *a lot* of hormones coursing through your body, which can make you feel justifiably insane. If the baby didn't physically come out of your tum-tum but you're the primary caregiver, you still have a myriad of intense hormones, emotions, concerns, thoughts, and more rushing through you. Cut yourself some freakin' slack and know that all those infamous blissful emotions will come with time.

- **Are you asking for expert help?** If you feel like something is off, beyond being tired and confused about how to navigate all the newness, call in support in the form of a therapist. They can help you determine if you're experiencing some postpartum blues (which can be soothed by the following suggestions), or if you're experiencing postpartum depression and need deeper help in the form of additional therapy and, potentially, medication. Nothing wrong with asking for help! The bravest among us are the best at asking for help.

- **Are you eating enough of the healthy stuff?** The food you put in your body has a dramatic effect on the dance of your hormones and mood. Make sure you're eating enough, and enough of the right stuff.

- **Are you drinking enough water?** If your body is shriveling up with dehydration, your emotions will act out. Drink a minimum of one hundred ounces of water per day, and take a long sip anytime you're feeling overwhelmed. Before you react to any negative stimuli, drink some water.

- **Are you moving around?** Physical activity releases endorphins, infuses you with fresh oxygen, and pulls you out of stagnation. Activity is good. Get up and move a bit. If you're the one who pushed a baby out of your petunia, you probably don't feel like running that 5k next weekend, or even walking to the mailbox, but a little shuffle to the kitchen for a banana will do you good. If you have explicit instructions from your care provider to stay in bed because of a C-section or other special circumstance, listen to them and focus on eating right, drinking plenty of water, and easing back into movement as soon as you get the green light.

- **Are you talking to someone over twelve months of age?** Talking can cleanse the soul. If you're feeling blue, talk it out. If you're feeling lost, talk it out. If you can't figure out which part is the front of the diaper, talk it out. Allowing yourself to verbally spit up on an empathetic fellow adult who will actively dole out loves, hugs, and words of advice (if requested) can make you feel like a rejuvenated "ready-for-baby-bonding" human again. Don't feel like you need to hide your sadness or your concerns about being a competent bonder. There's no shame in processing extreme change like a normal-feeling human.

Be gentle with your Self as you work (yes, sometimes it can feel like work) to find the sweet spot of bonding that works for you and your baby. It's a process that can happen over a long period of time, and it doesn't need to be instantaneous. And if you're reading this, it's proof that you're one rad mama who is committed to doing right by your baby and Self, even if it's really stinking hard to do sometimes!

Three Guiding Words

One key to bonding is releasing the stress conjured by all the tasks you "must" get through. One way to step out of this stress is to select three guiding words each day and, for the most part, take only those actions that sync with the messages of these words.

For example, my words today are *connect*, *write*, and *cleanse*. And this is how they'll guide me:

- **Connect:** I will be fully present, connecting with my child, my partner, and any other living creature I come into contact with, including myself. I will spread love, spread joy, let go of petty worries, and focus on what is important. I will make quality connections through quality interactions. I will connect to love.

- **Write:** I will spend three or more hours in a peaceful environment, entirely immersed in writing. I will remove phones, social media, and all other distractions. I will allow myself to focus only on writing and soaking in the value of words. (I also have a babysitter for three hours today.)

- **Cleanse:** I will cleanse my body of toxins by moving it and by preparing nourishing meals I can continue to feed my family for the rest of the week. I will spend an hour cleansing my home of unneeded objects that obstruct my ability to place focus on what I value. I will cleanse the poop from my child's diaper. And fine, I'll cleanse that disgusting space under the toilet.

My three-guiding-words practice hones my focus onto satisfying purposes and allows me to achieve value in each day. Instead of feeling overwhelmed by all the little stuff, I settle into the three main ideas I've committed to. Because I have grunt work that needs to be done, I ensure that it's also sprinkled into the words I select for each day. Since I started this practice, I've noticed that I move more slowly, yet get more done (and have more fun with my kiddo!).

How to Do It

Each evening, mindfully select the three words that will guide you the following day. (Or if your mental light is brightest in the morning, select your three words for the day before you get out of bed.) Write the words on a sticky note and post it in a prominent location. Look at the words frequently, and set the intention that they will inform your actions and thoughts that day. Allow the words to pull you out of petty stress.

Take a moment now to write your three words of intention for tomorrow.

Foster the Five Senses

If you're having trouble figuring out the best way to bond, focus on stimulating your baby's five senses, one at a time. First, focus on exciting Baby's sense of sight by showing her a striking image with bold colors, or taking her on a walk outside, frequently pausing to examine leaves or bark. Then, place your attention on rousing your baby's sense of smell by allowing her to smell a tissue with a few drops of a pleasant essential oil, like lavender or orange oil, or walk outside after your partner cuts the grass. Next, stimulate your baby's sense of touch by giving her a massage or cradling her to your body and gently stroking her scalp. Now it's time to awaken her sense of taste by allowing her to feed via breast or bottle. Finally, intrigue her sense of sound by singing a lulling song, or playing your favorite song.

Here are a few more sense-stimulating ideas:

- **Talk to Baby:** Chat about anything: the color of her poop, the 2008 financial meltdown, the best plan of attack for eating a funnel cake — whatever.
- **Sing to Baby:** Sing the tones loud and proud, even if you're deaf to them. Baby doesn't care.
- **Play with Baby:** Clean, hike, cook, drum, rattle stuff: your playtime does not need to be under the umbrella of traditional play; as long as you're doing something with your baby and communicating with her while doing it, she'll have a blast.

Motherhood can occasionally make you feel like a chunk of your brain was pulled out and thrown into the bushes, making it hard to figure out what the heck to do with the adorable little thing in your arms. One sense at a time, Mama, one sense at a time.

This bond you're forging is everlasting, causing you and your baby to release bursts of love hormones and love energy when you're together (or just thinking of one another). Even when your child turns into a teen who rolls her eyes and declines your phone calls, the love force will still be strong.

From My Heart to Yours

I was really bad at the whole "quality" aspect of bonding. I loved my baby and had fun staring at him, but then I would get bored, or feel like I needed to be doing some type A–level accomplishing. I felt guilty when I was with him because I felt like I needed to be working/creating, and I felt guilty when I was working/creating because I wasn't paying enough attention to him. Nothing "quality" got done. My bonding abilities were subpar, and my work creations were usually left yearning to be finished. And housekeeping … Ha!

Then, I decided to force myself to claim my choices. When I made the choice to bond, I fully stepped into that choice (with practice) — putting away my phone, going into a space that didn't have visual reminders of my non-baby to-dos, and being happy in knowing that the connecting I was doing with my baby was fostering the ultimate creation of my life: a well-loved human who thinks I am cool (sometimes). When I would make the choice to work, I would find a loving supporter to hang with my baby while I fully committed to work without regret. Value and satisfaction began seeping into my days.

— Bailey Gaddis, Ojai, California
(mama to sweet little Huddy Bear)

RIDDLE: How many words should you choose each day to set the intentions for your actions?

Go to **YourSereneLife.wordpress.com/chapter-twenty-three** and use the one-word riddle answer as your offer code to download the relaxation recording for this chapter!

CALL TO PLEASURE

- Choose three guiding words each day to clarify where to place your time. (Make sure one of them encourages quality time with your newborn; and one, quality time with your Self.)
- Find your favorite bonding rituals with your baby. Do you like to read to him? Sing to him? Stare at him? Make funny sounds at him? Explore the various ways you can bond, determining what you find enjoyable, and what you find boring. Bond the way you want to bond.

PARTING WISH

Let's talk about separation anxiety — not for you and baby, but for you and me! I'm attached to you now and don't want to say goodbye.

But you're so ready. We've gone through an epic journey together, and now it's time for you to go kick some parenting ass (or maybe just wipe it). My parting wish for you is that you continue to absorb all this information, throw out what doesn't resonate, marinate in all the *Yes!* moments you had in these pages, then go out and do what feels best for *you*. Allow all the juicy wisdom you've always had percolating in your mind-body-spirit shrine to continue to trickle (and sometimes blast) out of you, creating space for the ever-evolving goddess you are to continue stepping into her power and leading the charge.

You. Are. My. Hero.

xo,

Bailey

ACKNOWLEDGMENTS

I would like to line up the following people and give them each a long hug and non-creepy stare that says, "Thank you for sharing your awesomeness with me."

My son, Hudson — You ignited my passion for pregnancy, childbirth, and early motherhood and changed me in ways I didn't even know I wanted to change. I look forward to continuing to grow with you.

Eric, my cocreator of children, intimacy, joy, and laundry — You were like my doula during the many years it took me to birth this book, and your willingness to take on more than your fair share of the household duties while I holed up in my office to write makes me adore you in all ways.

Mom and Dad — The daily love you offer my little family is what created the space for me to craft this book without feeling guilty for abandoning said family for hours (sometimes days) at a time. And compliments to your mothers, Betty Gaddis Yndo and Anna Lucille Moore, for filling me with a knowingness that my voice matters, and should be shared.

My brothers, Rowan and Tiarnan — For preparing me for motherhood during your teen years, and helping me in motherhood by guiding Hudson through the tangled ropes of early childhood.

Lou and Gary — For always being willing to fill in the gaps with food, babysitting, and ever-present love.

Emily Heckman, my first editor and care provider for my words and ideas — Your spot-on wisdom and ability to bring eloquence to what I was trying to say gave me the confidence to move this book past conception into full-on gestation.

My literary agent, Paul Levine — For immediately seeing the value in my proposal and finding a home for it with my dream publisher.

Georgia Hughes, editorial director extraordinaire — Your ability to respect and support my vision, and know how to craft it into a book that clearly delivers the intended message, leaves me in awe of your talent. And to the rest of the New World Library team, your work is changing the world.

My copyeditor, Patricia Heinicke — Your intuitive feedback helped me transform *Feng Shui Mommy* from a book I was pretty pleased with to a publication I'm stoked to share with the mamas of the world. And bless you for your sensitivity!

Amanda Sandoval, my graphic design wizard — For taking my chaotic notes and birthing the exact images I was trying to describe. Magic.

John Phaneuf, the master of cinematic arts — For helping me encapsulate the essence of this book in a trailer that reminds me why I do what I do every time I watch it. I'll bet you never thought you'd know so much about placentas and breast milk — you're welcome.

Zhena Muzyka — For helping me trust that I had a message worth spreading, and championing my efforts through each phase. Your support, coupled with the mama-wisdom and "laugh till I pee a little bit" wit of Jessica Cauffiel, Sunne Justice, and Patrice Karst, made me feel less alone and more inspired on this often-solitary journey.

Robin Gerber — For reminding me that I was good enough, and to keep on keepin' on, even when I felt like I was locked in a room of dead ends.

Taryn Longo and the rest of my badass Ojai mama tribe — You give me daily reminders of what it looks like to mother with purpose, and you are quick with a warm embrace and the perfect words when I feel like I'm totally failing at all the things.

Raven and Sarah, and the Oak Grove early-childhood-sages Laurie, Emma, and Adrienne — You help care for Hudson with such loving intention and skill I feel like a better mother when I leave him in your guardianship.

Hugs, kisses, and even more hugs to you all.

NOTES

Chapter 1. Reclaiming Serenity

Page 16, *Doctors were forbidden to offer care to these women*: Marie Mongan, *Hypno-Birthing: The Mongan Method — A Natural Approach to a Safe, Easier, More Comfortable Birthing* (Deerfield Beach, FL: Health Communications, Inc., 2005), 38–39.

Page 16, *In "Navajo Ceremonial System," Leland C. Wyman explains that*: Leland C. Wyman, "Navajo Ceremonial System," in *Handbook of North American Indians*, vol. 10, *Southwest*, ed. Alfonso Ortiz, 539 (Washington, D.C.: Smithsonian Institution, 1983), http://www.uscis.humboldt.edu/jwpowell/Leland WymanHONAI-NavajoCeremonialSystem,reduced.pdf.

Chapter 2. Feng Shui

Page 27, *Because NASA is all about bringing people back to Earth*: Anne Johnson and Keith Bounds, "Interior Landscape Plants for Indoor Air Pollution Abatement," *NASA* (September 15, 1989): 9–13, https://ntrs.nasa.gov/archive/nasa /casi.ntrs.nasa.gov/19930073077.pdf.

Chapter 5. The Nourishing Basics

Page 67, *According to a study published in the* Journal of Obstetrics and Gynecology: Oqba Al-Kuran, Lama Al-Mehaisen, Hiba Bawadi, Soha Beitawi, and Zouhair Amarin, "The Effect of Late Pregnancy Consumption of Date Fruit on Labour and Delivery," *Journal of Obstetrics and Gynecology* 31, no. 1 (2011): 29–31.

Chapter 7. Creating the Birth Sanctuary

Page 89, *Here are a few fun stats found in the* Cochrane Reviews: E. D. Hodnett, S. Gates, G. J. Hofmeyr, C. Sakala, and J. Weston, "Continuous Support for Women during Childbirth," *Cochrane Database of Systemic Reviews*, 2012, Issue 10, Art. No.: CD003766, https://www.ncbi.nlm.nih.gov/pubmed/21328263.

Chapter 8. Birth Preferences

Page 102, *A study by the American Society of Anesthesiologists has shown*: American Society of Anesthesiologists (ASA), "Most Healthy Women Would Benefit from Light Meal during Labor," *ScienceDaily*, October 25, 2015, www.science daily.com/releases/2015/10/151025010725.htm.

Page 106, *According to the* American Journal of Obstetrics & Gynecology: Amy M. Romano, "Research Summaries for Normal Birth," *Journal of Perinatal Education* 14, no. 2 (Spring 2005): 52–55 (doi: 10.1624/105812405X44745).

Page 107, *These skin-to-skin benefits are believed to have*: Dr. William Sears, "Ask Dr. Sears: Co-Sleeping a SIDS Danger?" *Parenting*, November 2011, http://www.parenting.com/article/ask-dr-sears-co-sleeping-a-sids-danger.

Page 107, *Mom's chances of hemorrhaging are neither heightened nor lessened*: S. J. McDonald, P. Middleton, T. Dowswell, and P. S. Morris, "Effect of Timing of Umbilical Cord Clamping of Term Infants on Maternal and Neonatal Outcomes," *Cochrane Database of Systematic Reviews*, 2013, Issue 7, Art. No.: CD004074 (doi: 10.1002/14651858.CD004074.pub3).

Chapter 9. Nontraditional Pregnancy

Page 119, *A study of California parents, "Strategies for Disclosure: How Parents Approach Telling Their Children That They Were Conceived with Donor Gametes"*: K. MacDougall, G. Becker, J. Scheib, and R. Nachtigall, *Fertility and Sterility* 87, no. 3 (2007): 524–33.

Chapter 10. Water, Water, Water — and, Oh Yeah, Water!

Page 124, *In 1994, Dr. Masaru Emoto and a team of researchers observed*: Masaru Emoto, "What Is the Photograph of Frozen Water Crystals?" *Welcome to the World of Water*, 2010, http://www.masaru-emoto.net/english/water-crystal.html.

Chapter 16. Birthing Positions and Light Touch Healing

Page 203, *Smart people at the Touch Research Institute reported*: T. Field, M. Hernandez-Reif, S. Taylor, O. Quintino, and I. Burman (Touch Research

Institute, University of Miami School of Medicine), "Labor Pain Is Reduced by Massage Therapy," *Journal of Psychosomatic Obstetrics and Gynecology* 18, no. 4 (1997): 286–91.

Page 203, *And not all touch is equal — another study found that moms found massage*: Elizabeth R. Birch, "The Experience of Touch Received during Labor," *Journal of Nurse-Midwifery* 31, no. 6 (November–December 1986): 270–75.

Chapter 20. Breastfeeding

Page 234, *A study done by the National Institute of Environmental Health Sciences showed*: Carolyn Davis Cockey, "Breastfeeding Decreases Infant Mortality," *AWHONN Lifelines* 8, no. 4 (August–September 2004): 306, http://nwh journal.org/article/S1091-5923(15)31152-3/pdf.

Page 234, *In addition, a large German study published in 2009 found*: M. M. Vennemann, T. Bajanowski, B. Brinkmann, G. Jorch, K. Yücesan, C. Sauerland, and E. A. Mitchell, "Does Breastfeeding Reduce the Risk of Sudden Infant Death Syndrome?" *Pediatrics* 123, no. 3 (2009): e406–410, http://www.ncbi.nlm.nih.gov/pubmed/19254976 (doi: 10.1542/peds.2008 -2145).

Page 234, *A study published in the journal* JAMA Pediatrics *found*: M. B. Belfort, S. L. Rifas-Shiman, K. P. Kleinman, et al., "Infant Feeding and Childhood Cognition at Ages 3 and 7 Years: Effects of Breastfeeding Duration and Exclusivity," *JAMA Pediatrics* 167, no. 9 (2013): 836–44, http://archpedi .jamanetwork.com/article.aspx?articleid=1720224 (doi: 10.1001/jamapediatrics .2013.455).

Page 235, *Your body then responds by creating custom milk*: Laura Sanders, "Backwash from Nursing Babies May Trigger Infection Fighters," *ScienceNews*, September 15, 2015, www.sciencenews.org/blog/growth-curve/backwash-nursing-babies -may-trigger-infection-fighters.

RECOMMENDED RESOURCES

Following is the list of resources I offer to clients.

Midwife Associations

American College of Nurse-Midwives (Midwifc.org)
Midwives Alliance of North America (MANA.org)
National Association of Certified Professional Midwives (NACPM.org)
The North American Registry of Midwives (NARM.org)

Doula Resources

American Pregnancy Association, "Having a Doula: Is a Doula for Me?"
    (AmericanPregnancy.org/labor-and-birth/having-a-doula)
DONA International (DONA.org/what-is-a-doula/find-a-doula)
DoulaMatch.net
Your Serene Life, "Birth Doula Services" (YourSereneLife.wordpress.com/birth
    -doula-services)

Childbirth Preparation

Birthing from Within (BirthingFromWithin.com)
Bradley Method of Husband-Coached Natural Childbirth (BradleyBirth.com)
Complete Guide to the Alexander Technique (alexandertechnique.com)
HypnoBirthing Institute (US.HypnoBirthing.com)
Lamaze International (Lamaze.org)

Your Serene Life, "Feng Shui Mommy Online Childbirth Course" (YourSerene
    Life.wordpress.com/online-course)

Feng Shui Resources

About.com, "Feng Shui" (FengShui.about.com)

Bailey Gaddis, "The Feng Shui–Inspired Nursery," YouTube video (YouTube.com
    /watch?v=UgToPorCDWU)

Cathleen McCandless, *Feng Shui That Makes Sense: Easy Ways to Create a Home
    That Feels as Good as It Looks* (Minneapolis, MN: Two Harbors Press, 2011)

Marie Kondo, *The Life-Changing Magic of Tidying Up: The Japanese Art of De-
    cluttering and Organizing* (Berkeley, CA: Ten Speed Press, 2014)

Baby Proofing Resources

BabyCenter, "Childproofing Checklist: Before Your Baby Crawls" (Baby
    Center.com/0_childproofing-checklist-before-your-baby-crawls_9446.bc)

Parents Magazine website, "Babyproofing" (Parents.com/baby/safety/baby
    proofing)

Relaxation and Hypnosis Recordings

Your Serene Life, "Breech Turn Hypnosis Recording" (https://YourSereneLife
    .wordpress.com/breech-turn-hypnosis-recording)

Your Serene Life, "Guided Relaxation Downloads" (YourSereneLife.wordpress.com
    /relaxation-downloads)

Nutrition and Exercise

American Pregnancy Association, "Placenta Encapsulation" (AmericanPregnancy
    .org/first-year-of-life/placental-encapsulation)

FitPregnancy.com, "Guide to Drinking Tea during Pregnancy" (FitPregnancy.com
    /nutrition/prenatal-nutrition/tea-time)

FitPregnancy.com, "Recipes" (FitPregnancy.com/nutrition/recipes)

TheBump.com, "Best Pregnancy Workout DVDs" (TheBump.com/a/pregnancy
    -workout-dvds)

INDEX

Page references given in *italics* indicate
illustrations or material contained in
their captions.

abdominal pressure, 178
abdominal strengthening, 221
acupressure, 141
acupuncture, 138, 141
air, fresh: bedroom organization and, 167,
   168–69, 175; feng shui and, 26, 28, 33–34;
   walking for, 54–55
alcohol, 67
alone time: activities for, 228–29; breathing
   exercise, 225; Call to Pleasure checklist,
   232; From Her Heart to Yours, 231; minimum amount of, 227–28; mother-baby
   bonding and, 269–70; partner and,
   229–30; riddle, 232; scheduling strategies
   and, 230–31; self-love and, 225–26; sense
   of Self and, 226–27
American Academy of Pediatrics, 235
American Journal of Obstetrics & Gynecology,
   106
American Society of Anesthesiologists, 102
amnesia, 185
amniotic fluid, 105, 123

amygdala, 71
anaerobic exercise, 208
animals, birthing instincts of, 23–24
ankles, 123
antibiotics, 134
antioxidants, 62, 63
anxiety, 123
aquatic meditation, 55
artificial nipples, 243
artwork, 34, 126, 175, 220
ATP (adenosine triphosphate), 208
attachment, releasing, 220
audiobooks, 48, 54

baby: bedroom organization and, 167–68;
   "being the baby," 126; brain development
   of, 267; breastfeeding and, 233, 234–35;
   breech baby, 137–38; descent of, 104–5,
   177; emergence of, 105–6, 184–87; energy
   nook for, 172, 175; ideal position of, *197*,
   197; massaging, 262; movements of, 113;
   packing list for, 86; postpartum care,
   106–8; repositioning of, 103; scent of,
   266; sleep sounds of, 260–61; stimulating
   senses of, 274–75; water as percentage of,
   122; "wearing," 268

cancer, 63, 236

carbon dioxide, 206

care provider: birth preferences and, 97–98, 112; birth sanctuary choice and, 82; home births and, 87; pain relief and, 138–39; postpartum body changes and, 248, 250, 251, 252, 253; resistance from, 97; special circumstances and, 131, 135, 136, 144; station numbers used by, *177*, 177–78; water births and, 127–28

carnival foods, 67

Cauffiel, Jessica, 17–18

cervix dilation, 99, 101, 177–78, 182–83

cesarean birth: attitude shift toward, 141–42; birth preferences regarding, 98, 109–10; birth stories of, 20; childbirthing fear and, 15; doulas and decreased rates of, 89; emotions involved in, 141; expectations of, 141; From Her Heart to Yours, 142–43; hospital choice and, 83; premature birth as result of, 135

chakra system, 216–18, 222. *See also* sacral chakra

chi (energy; life force), 3–4, 34, 36

childbirthing: ancient view of, 16, 19; animal instincts and, 23–24; author's experience, xv–xix, 1–2; books on, 1; breathing exercises, xiii, 13; Call to Pleasure checklist, 9, 25; curiosity about, 6; divided opinions about, 5–6; focal point during, 93; HypnoBirthing, 1–2; premature, 135–37; preparation resources, 285–86; riddles, 9, 24; rituals of, 21–22, 25; stories of, 19–20, 25; support network for, 6, 22–23; touch during, 199–203, 204; unpredictability of, 176. *See also* fear of childbirthing/ pregnancy; pregnancy

childbirth preparation classes, 120–21

childhood leukemia, 233

children's books, 120

chiropractic, 141

cigarettes, 67

cleaning supplies, 173

clothes storage, 171–72

clutter, 26, 29, 34, 167, 168, 173, 175

Cochrane Reviews, 89, 107

coconut water, 92, 102, 124

colors, 26, 31–33, 34, 167, 169, 175

colostrum, 235

Commission for the Accreditation of Birth Centers, 83

complications, 130, 131. *See also* special circumstances

constipation, 257

cooing, 267

cord clamping, 107

cord stump care, 259

cosleeping, 107, 260

courage, 75

cradle hold (breastfeeding position), 239

cramping, 136, 178

crane, 93

cravings, 228–29

creativity, 18–19, 25, 34, 172, 219–20

crown chakra, 218

crystals, 168–69

C-sections. *See* cesarean birth

cuddling, 267–68

dancing, 48–49, 140, 221, 267

dates (fruit), 67, 140

deep breathing, 183–84; author's experience, 181; for baby repositioning, 103; benefits of, 205–9; breathing exercise, 205; Descent Breathing, 211–12, 215; De-stressor Breathing, 211, 214, 215; in everyday life, 205; fear release through, 72; FTP syndrome relieved by, 210–14; From Her Heart to Yours, 214; during labor, 179, 181; Labor Breathing, 211, 214, 215; oxygen and, 206–9; as pain relief, 45, 124; during perineal massage, 212–13; riddle, 214

dehydration, 102

depression, 73

Descent Breathing, 211–12, 215

De-stressor Breathing, 211, 214, 215
diabetes, 133. *See also* gestational diabetes
diaper rash, 258–59
diarrhea, 178, 257
dietary restrictions, 67–68
distractions, 179, 242–43
distress, levels of, 36–37
donations, 174
doulas, 285. *See also* birth doula; postpartum
   doula
dressing needs, 171–72

earth element, 3, 4
earth hues, 93
egg donors, 113, 115–16, 118–19
Egypt, ancient, 23, 24
electronics, 172–73, 175
Emotional Freedom Technique (EFT),
   35–39, *38*, 43
emotions: confused, during labor, 178,
   185–86; fear-related, liberation of, 73–75,
   77; with PLR, 157–58; with premature
   birth, 135; triggering of, 74; with unplanned pregnancy, 132
Emoto, Masaru, 124
empathy, 271
endorphins, 45, 54, 67, 199–200
energizing side-angle pose, *50*, 50
energy nooks, 167, 170–73, 175
engorgement, 237–38
epidurals, 20, 89, 98, 138
essential oils, 92
exercise, prenatal: attitude shift toward,
   45–46; author's experience, 44; benefits
   of, 45; breathing exercise, 44; for breech
   turn, 138; Call to Pleasure checklist, 58;
   From Her Heart to Yours, 57; Kegels,
   56–57, 58; for natural induction, 140;
   precautions before, 45, 46, 49–50, 58;
   pre-pregnancy routines and, 46–47;
   "quickie" suggestions, 47–49, 58;
   resources, 286; riddle, 57; swimming,
   55–56, 58; visualizing, 46; walking, 54–55,
   58; yoga, 49–54, *50–54*, 58

exercise equipment, 173, 175
external cephalic version (ECV) procedure,
   138
eye contact, 229, 270

face masks, 110
family, explaining nontraditional pregnancy
   to, 117–18, 121
family practitioners, 87
fast food, 67
fat burning, 208–9
fear of childbirthing/pregnancy: about
   baby care, 255; cultural images of, 14–15;
   cultural origins of, 16; as dread of the
   unknown, 176; giving voice to, 73; liberating, 73–75, 77; listing sources of, 25;
   mind-body effects of, 71; misconceptions
   about, 70–71; OBGYN consultation and
   soothing of, 87; special circumstances
   and, 130; stress produced by, 71; sympathetic nervous system and, 72
fear release: author's experience, 74–75;
   breathing exercise, 70; Call to Pleasure
   checklist, 77; through creativity, 18–19,
   through EFT, 35–39; emotions liberated
   for, 73; From Her Heart to Yours, 76;
   ninety-second release, 73, 77; riddle, 76;
   sympathetic/parasympathetic nervous
   systems and, 71, 72–73
fear-tension-pain (FTP) syndrome, 210
feng shui: for bedroom organization, 167,
   168–69; benefits of, 26; breathing exercise, 26; Call to Pleasure checklist, 33–34;
   colors for, 26, 31–33, 34; decluttering for,
   26, 29, 34; defined, 3; five elements in,
   3–4; focal point choices, 93; fresh air for,
   26, 28, 33–34; From Her Heart to Yours,
   30–31; lighting for, 26, 29–31, 34; plants
   for, 26, 27–28, 33; pregnancy and distur-
   bance of, 14; resources, 286; riddle, 33
Feng Shui Mommy, 3–4
fiber, 62, 63–64, 66, 69, 249
fire element, 3, 4

first sign of labor to-do list, 94

first trimester. *See* exercise, prenatal; fear of childbirthing/pregnancy; fear release; feng shui; nontraditional healing; nutrition; pregnancy

fish oil, 65, 66

flexibility, 231

fluorescent lights, 30

focal point, 93

folate, 62

folder, birth, 112

folic acid, 62, 64

forceps-assisted births, 89, 105

formulas, poop from, 257

forward lean, 195, *195*

fountains, 28

fourth trimester. *See* alone time; baby care; breastfeeding; mother-baby bonding; postpartum body

fried foods, 67

friends: explaining nontraditional pregnancy to, 117–18, 121

From Her Heart to Yours: alone time, 231; baby care, 263; birthing positions, 204; birth sanctuary, 94–95; breastfeeding, 244; cesarean birth, 142–43; deep breathing, 214; fear release, 76; feng shui, 30–31; how to use, 8–9; labor, 188–89; mother-baby bonding, 275; nutrition, 68; postpartum body, 253–54; pregnancy, 17–18; prenatal exercise, 57; sacral chakra, 221–22; self-hypnosis, 153–54; water births, 128–29

fruits, 63, 66, 69, 93

furniture arrangement, 167, 173–74

furniture storage, 170

Gaddis, Bailey, 76, 221–22, 231, 275

gas-relieving child's pose, *54*, 54

gestational diabetes, 61, 63, 133–34

gestational surrogates, 113, 116–17, 118, 119–20

gifts, 125

glycogen, 208–9

grains, 64, 66, 69

gratitude, 108–9, 124, 141–42

gravity, 191

green (color), 33

green foods, 62, 66, 69

grief, 115

Grotto of Massabielle (France), 125

Group B strep, 74–75; 134

gum disease, 136

hair loss, 247, 250

handbag hold (breastfeeding position), 240

hands and knees (birthing position), *196–97*, 196–97

happiness, 207

health insurance, 82

heartburn, 178

heart chakra, 217–18

hemorrhaging, 106

hemorrhoids, 123, 247, 249–50

hep-locks, 99–100

hetero-hypnosis, 149–50, 154

Hinduism, 49

hip squeeze, *202*, 202

holism, 14

home, repurposing, 48

home birthing kits, 92

home births, 5; care provider and, 87; checklist for, 93–94; lactation consultants for, 240–41; necessities for, 86, 91–93; selection considerations, 82–83; space selection for, 89–91

hormonal surges, 247

hospitals: birth preferences for, 99–101; home births and, 87; packing lists for, 84–86; selection considerations, 82–84

houseplants, 26, 27–28, 33

hypertension, 137

HypnoBirthing, 1–2

hypnosis: author's experience, 146; breathing exercise, 145; defined, 145–46; everyday states of, 146; experience of, 149; holistic effects of, 146; misconceptions about, 147; negative/positive swap in, 150–51;

ABOUT THE AUTHOR

Bailey Gaddis, C.Ht., HBCE, is an author and contributor to *Working Mother*, *Pregnancy and Newborn*, Disney's *Babble*, *The Huffington Post*, *Cosmopolitan*, *Redbook*, *Expectful*, *Elephant Journal*, *Scary Mommy*, and other publications that are into her style of weaving words. She continuously finds inspiration for her writing via the stream of consciousness flowing out of her son's mouth, and the insane shenanigans she witnesses during births (and at the park before nap time).

Her work as a childbirth preparation educator, birth doula, hypnotherapist, amateur smoothie chef, and past egg donor and surrogacy coordinator allows her to work with rockstar pregnant women and their gorgeous offspring every day. She's fairly certain "new baby smell" is the most enticing aroma on Earth.

When she's not supporting a woman in a squat and urging her to "breathe that baby down," Bailey enjoys digging in the dirt with her son while attempting to avoid the clumps he occasionally flings at her hair, and trying to figure out the context of his (usually) coherent babbling. She fancies herself a holistically hippie Taurean with an unfortunate proclivity for reality television, sugar, and tie-dye — all at the same time.

She lives every day in complete awe of the creation, birth, and nurturing of new life, and considers the mother-baby bond the pinnacle of magic, which is why she's thinking about beginning to think about Baby Number Two.

For a list of Bailey's online courses, visit **BaileyGaddis.com**.

NEW WORLD LIBRARY is dedicated to publishing books and other media that inspire and challenge us to improve the quality of our lives and the world.

We are a socially and environmentally aware company. We recognize that we have an ethical responsibility to our customers, our staff members, and our planet.

We serve our customers by creating the finest publications possible on personal growth, creativity, spirituality, wellness, and other areas of emerging importance. We serve New World Library employees with generous benefits, significant profit sharing, and constant encouragement to pursue their most expansive dreams.

As a member of the Green Press Initiative, we print an increasing number of books with soy-based ink on 100 percent postconsumer-waste recycled paper. Also, we power our offices with solar energy and contribute to non-profit organizations working to make the world a better place for us all.

Our products are available in bookstores everywhere.

www.newworldlibrary.com

At NewWorldLibrary.com you can download our catalog,
subscribe to our e-newsletter, read our blog,
and link to authors' websites, videos, and podcasts.

Find us on Facebook, follow us on Twitter, and watch us on YouTube.

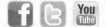

Send your questions and comments our way!
You make it possible for us to do what we love to do.

Phone: 415-884-2100 or 800-972-6657
Catalog requests: Ext. 10 | Orders: Ext. 10 | Fax: 415-884-2199
escort@newworldlibrary.com

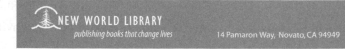

NEW WORLD LIBRARY
publishing books that change lives   14 Pamaron Way, Novato, CA 94949